COLUMBIA COLLEGE
371.102R826F   C1   V 0
THE FORBIDDEN APPLE$ PALM SPRINGS   CA

3 2711 00002 7029

CO-AUL-499

371.102 R826f

Ross, Victor J., 19

The forbidden apple

The Forbidden Apple

Dedication

For Jerome Cramer and Richard Hostrop

DISCARD
the forbidden apple

Sex in the Schools

by
Victor J. Ross and John Marlowe

LIBRARY
OF
COLUMBIA COLLEGE
CHICAGO, ILLINOIS

An 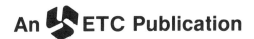 ETC Publication

Library of Congress Cataloging in Publication Data

Ross, Victor J., 1935-
The Forbidden Apple

1. Teacher-student relationships. 2. Child molesting.
3. Sexual harassment. 4. Sexual deviation.
5. Homosexuality.
I. Marlowe, John, 1938- . II. Title.
LB1033.R675 1985   371.1'02   84-6152
ISBN 0-88280-107-4

No part of this publication may be reproduced or transmitted in any form or by any means, electronic or mechanical, including photocopy, recording, or any information storage and retrieval system known or to be invented, without permission in writing from the publisher, except by a reviewer who wishes to quote brief passages in connection with a review written for inclusion in a magazine, periodical, newspaper, or broadcast.

Copyright © 1985 by Victor J. Ross, Jr. and John Marlowe

Published by ETC Publications
Palm Springs
California 92263-1608

Printed in the United States of America

All rights reserved

371.102 R826f

Ross, Victor J., 1935-

The forbidden apple

CONTENTS

Introduction

Let's talk, shall we? Let's have a little chat about teachers 'in love' with students.

"Don't walk away. Don't assume this is written to be sensational, to shock you, to anger you, or to offend you. Your assumption would be wrong.

". . . (We) write this because it is needed."

* * *

In one sense, the quotation above — the first six sentences of an article entitled "The Broken Taboo: What You Can Do When Teachers Get Too Cozy With Their Students," which appeared in the March, 1981 issue of *The Executive Educator* magazine — led to the development of this book. The story detailed several incidents where teachers became romantically and sexually involved with their students, and provided guidelines to administrators about how to deal with them. It brought a sensitive and very real problem out of the closet and dealt with relationships few in education care to acknowledge. Reader response was strong and positive. Readers said that these indiscretions happen in education and administrators have to do something about them; help is needed.

That's one reason for this book, one explanation for why it was written.

There's another very compelling reason for proceeding with the book. Simply stated, it is this: in every instance, a bite of the forbidden apple creates a victim. Even when the bite is imaginary. Even when there is no case — the child's accusation of molestation or harrassment proves to be of no substance — even then, there is a victim, there are repercussions that often inflict permanent damage.

For example, an acquaintance of the authors, a superintendent who agreed to assist in the research for this book, tells us of a teacher who was accused of taking liberties with a student. The charges were untrue. The superintendent got a confession from the student that the entire story had been concocted to gain revenge for an 'unfair' grade. However, after the superintendent resolved the problem, it refused to go away. Parents continued to circulate rumors; school board members wanted to know why the young man was still employed when it was clear he was preying on young children for sexual favors. After more than a year of battling the absurd irrationalities, the superintendent, still convinced of the teacher's innocence, counseled him to resign. It was a small community, and it was painfully clear that the young man would never overcome the situation. He resigned, an innocent victim of not so innocent sexual harrassment, and moved away.

We all know, further, that the victims of *real* indiscretion also suffer.

Therefore, while this book deals with a taboo, it deals with something we all know really happens. We all want to know what, if anything, can be done about it. The topic needs to be aired, explored, and analyzed. That's what this book is all about.

It has not been an easy assignment. First, there is no research or literature of any substance, no wealth of empirical data, on the problem of sex in the schools. Seeking out cases, obtaining interviews, soliciting opinions — all this has been somewhat akin to ghost-hunting. At first it appears to be an impossible mission because no one wants to admit they believe in ghosts or have encountered a poltergeist. But, we discovered that when we were patient, serious, and understanding, and when we assured interviewees that data would be handled sensitively and for good purpose, people began to talk, documentation became possible. They told us about their encounters with a 'ghost:' sex in the schools.

A final point. Nearly all persons who contributed case histories for this book requested anonymity. That's understandable, and the reader needs to know that their requests have been respected. But it also needs to be understood that every incident described in this book is real. Each one has been written to protect the identity of those involved, but the authenticity has been documented. The alterations are minimal — a change in geographic location or grade level or a reversal of the sexes of the aggressor and victim — but the alterations are intentional, just as the cases are real.

The book is intended to benefit teachers, students, parents, and administrators who want to gain insights and guidelines for dealing with sexual exploitation and harrassment when they are faced with the problems.

Victor J. Ross
Aurora, Colorado

John Marlowe
San Francisco, California

About the Authors

Victor J. Ross and John Marlowe are both seasoned school administrators with a good deal in common. Ross, associate superintendent for instruction with the Aurora (Colorado) Public Schools, was a high school principal for ten years; Marlowe is a high school principal at present in California. Both men were selected by *The Executive Educator* magazine, a publication of the National School Boards Association, for recognition as one of the Top 100 Executive Educators in North America; Marlowe was honored in 1981, Ross in 1984.

Both are prolific free lance writers of fiction and non-fiction, and their works appear regularly in many national journals and magazines.

Ross began his writing career in earnest by authoring a novel about his experiences as a principal. The work of fiction, *Bite the Wall*, has been widely acclaimed for its pace and authentic realism. The novel was released in 1985 and was also published by ETC Publications.

Ross earned his B.A. and M.A. degrees at the University of Denver, the doctorate in education administration at the University of Colorado, and he lives with his wife and three children in Aurora, a suburb of Mile High Denver.

*   *   *

Marlowe started his education career as a substitute in San Francisco and is now principal of Albany High, which is in a small community next to Berkeley, California. He has lived and worked in various parts of Northern California and Athens, Greece. He was the recipient of a Fulbright-Hayes Travel-Study grant, and, like Ross, his articles, book reviews and fiction have appeared in many publications. He won the Charles Stewart Mott Award for his education writing, and he is an art critic for several publications on the West and East Coasts, an unlikely field of endeavor for a high school principal.

He has taught high school and college and most recently has moved back to San Francisco into a house on Russian Hill with his wife, daughter and son. Like everyone else in that city he is also working on a screenplay.

* * *

The manuscript was developed entirely by correspondence, with a few telephone calls now and then to check details. Obviously, the two authors got along well on the project, and the harmony was due in part to their admiration for one another's work.

Together, Marlowe and Ross have produced a valuable book on a sensitive topic that is both informative and very readable.

Prologue: Is It Safe?

Throughout the course of *The Forbidden Apple* readers will find two recurring themes. The first is that it appears very evident that sexual abuse and violent intimidation of children in school is on the increase. Another frequently presented premise is that schools must be safe places for youngsters.

We expect no one will argue very seriously about either idea by the time the book is finished.

While we didn't actually count them, unfortunately the authors had no trouble finding hundreds of incidents of sexual abuse in North America's schools, many more than we had occasion to use as examples in this book. Fair enough? It was our experience that sex-in-the-schools happens in tragic numbers, and we have included countless "Case Studies" in our presentation of problems and recommended solutions.

Consider then, that between the time the manuscript was submitted for typesetting and the time the camera-ready proof pages were returned by the publisher for editing and corrections two months later, at least three additional sex scandals of major and shocking proportions occurred.

In Nebraska officials were forced to close the state's school for the deaf and blind in order to investigate sex crimes against the children that, according to one investigator, seemed to involve the majority of adults — teachers and staff members — at the institution.

In nearby Colorado, parents of school children in Denver and its surrounding suburbs reached a state of near-panic when in a two-week period five children on their way to school were snatched by strangers and sexually molested. One girl was raped and murdered, her body discovered a few days later in the mountains near Nederland, Colorado.

The Colorado incidents did not occur at school, true, but all the victims were children on the way to school. Therefore, the majority of Denver area school districts have instituted the practice of calling the parents of every child absent to find out if they are really home ill. In the event this cannot be verified, foul play is presumed and police are called immediately.

Finally, in sunny Manhattan Beach, California, seven adults — the entire staff of the Virginia McMartin Pre-School — were indicted for sex abuse. The district attorney's office, according to the prosecutor in charge, had evidence that the school's founder and its six staff members committed 397 sex charges against children two to six years of age. *One Hundred Fifteen* specific offenses were documented in the indictment.

Manhattan Beach law officials interviewed over 200 children in preparing the case, and ninety per cent of the youngsters documented sex abuse, including pornography and lurid photographs.

The prosecutor, in presenting the case to the judge, was quoted as saying: ". . . it is abundantly clear that the horrors of what we have learned to date of what has occurred at that nursery school have effected an entire generation of children."

As one girl at the school told her mother, "Mom, a good day at school was a day when Ray (one of the staff members) would leave us alone."

* * *

Schools should be safe places for children. And adults, for that matter. Far too many of them are not.

Sex crimes at the school site should *not* be increasing, but the evidence indicates strongly that they *are*.

It is our deep and sincere hope that this book will contribute to the reduction of sex abuse in schools and at the same time present suggestions that will make all our schools what they must be: *safe*.

—JM & VJR

Chapter 1

Don't Stand So Close to Me

A careful attempt has been made to organize and categorize the instances of sex problems encountered in the schools — particularly the kindergarten through twelfth grade public schools — to present the essential details of incidents that fit in one of those categories or another, and to give the reader some guidelines that appear to be useful in similar situations he or she may come up against. No apologies for the effort to organize/ categorize/ and guideline the morass of problems. It represents the best format the writers could devise and it works about as well as any.

The curious reader has already skimmed ahead and is aware that in subsequent chapters the "why" is a question that is examined — *why* do teachers and educators violate the mores of society, the social contract, and break the taboo?

Readers may know too that the final chapter in this book represents a serious effort to organize all the guidelines and steps presented throughout the book and give some step-by-step advice worth knowing and following.

With this chapter, however, we won't worry about guidelines. We won't try to critique each of the events described. We will plain-and-simple present one man's roller coaster ride through a decade as a school principal, what he careened into and how often, and what he thought about it, and then at the end we'll make a couple of observations and speculations about the growth and development, as well as the real and the ideal, of this mucky problem called sex in the schools.

Chapter One represents a fast ride. Get ready for the who-what-when-where-how-and-why in rapid succession, (recognizing that the who is disguised, the what is basic reality, the when and where have been doctored, the how is clear, and the why will be dealt with later).

1

* * *

Jerry Fuller walked into his first principalship at the age of thirty. The year was 1968 and his master's degree and administrator credential were shiny new in their frames as he organized and personalized the trappings of his office at Kennedy Junior High School in a midwestern suburb.

Kennedy had a few problems with loose student discipline and a staff that was a bit on the youthful side and not entirely enamored with their assignment as teachers of the "storm and stress" age student, but all in all the problems were not insurmountable. Jerry Fuller was and is a fairly charismatic leader, a good curriculum man, and a great fan of the adolescent youngster. Things went well at Kennedy Junior High during Fuller's three-year tenure as its principal. Discipline problems all but disappeared, a popular activity program was introduced, and annual test scores showed improvement every year.

"I remember my three years at Kennedy with pride, with satisfaction," Fuller said, "but there's always that dark cloud hanging over it all. That's part of the memory too."

The dark cloud? It was comprised of three serious problems Fuller had to resolve. The first was a male teacher who had cultivated a sexual appetite for a ninth-grade girl. Fuller was able to obtain testimony from the girl, complete support from her parents, and with the backing of his superintendent he forced a resignation from the teacher.

"I guess I handled it well, but it was an ugly experience, and very hard on the emotions. It more or less shattered me to find that a teacher could do something like that," Fuller said. "I guess I was pretty naive then. And it really flattened me to find out a year later that the guy went directly to California and got a job teaching. No one ever made a reference call about him."

If Jerry Fuller was naive in his rookie year as a principal, he overcame it quickly and perhaps a bit too rudely. The second and third problems occurred almost simultaneously in Fuller's second year at Kennedy.

Several of his students — girls, for the most part — became runaways who couldn't resist the call of the hippie culture passing through town on its way to mecca: San Francisco's Haight Ashbury.

"Our kids — some of them, anyway — were really vulnerable to the lure of these drug-peddling pan-handling members of the hippie counter culture, or whatever the hell it was," Fuller said. "I got involved when our juvenile probation officer, a good friend of mine, told me where most the girls were going. He said the police were almost helpless to do anything; there were just too many kids passing through to try to sort out the local runaways."

Fuller brooded about the problem for nearly a week before deciding to get far more involved than is normally expected of a school principal. "I decided if the police couldn't find my girls and return them to their parents, maybe I could."

Fuller, his assistant principal, and the probation officer got in their car one evening, drove to the rapidly deteriorating section of the core city where the hippies-passing-through and their groupies tended to congregate, and started looking. "We checked a few old houses and had no luck," said Fuller, "so we decided to try a cafe that was supposed to be a prime hangout for these creeps."

It was. Fuller related that he never felt more uncomfortable or out of place in his life than when he and his two friends walked into the Starlight Coffee Shop. "Marijuana smoke was thick. You could smell the sweat and grubbiness of these bearded kids . . . it was a scene out of Dante's hell, as far as I'm concerned. And talk about feeling almost intimidated by the surly stares of these people. Three clean-shaven, middle-aged men wearing slacks and blazers fit in that environment about as well as . . . well, about like three cops walking in on a private stag show.

"But three of our girls from Kennedy, not one of them more than fifteen years old, were there, and we got them out and safely home, in spite of their protests. All were borderline starvation cases, all had hepatitis, all had pan-handled for food money without much success, all had been raped or gang-raped and tripped out of LSD and amphetamines and god knows what else."

While Jerry Fuller agreed that the abuse and degradation of junior high girls did not technically fall into the category of sex in the school's problems, he believes that what happend to American youth in the late Sixties and early Seventies did indeed have a negative impact on adults, and that it became a contributing factor to the increase in sex in the schools.

"I may be all wet, but I really believe that our inabilities to prevent or stop these crimes warped us. Youthful drug addicts preyed on teenagers, committed criminal acts, and got off with no punishment, by and large,'' Fuller said. ''For example, when the third problem — the third part of the dark cloud that hangs over my Kennedy memories — when it happened, I'll always remember one statement the offending teacher made.

''I had called him into my office to tell him I wanted his resignation or I was going to can him. He had just committed his third offense; he had been seen patting a student on her bottom and putting his hand up her blouse. 'God, Mr. Fuller,' the guy said, 'I admit it was wrong, but you know we were just teasing around. You want to fire me for it. What about all those hippies who screwed girls from this school and shot them all full of drugs. What happened to any of them? *Nothing*, that's what. I lose my job for an act of poor judgment, and that bunch literally gets away with murder.' ''

Fuller has a point. It may not be valid, but from his perspective — and based on his subsequent experiences — there is a logic behind his belief that sexual abuse in the schools has increased in direct proportion to the decrease or decline in our legal system's ability to deal justly with those who break the law.

''We've become cynical,'' Fuller said. ''Blame it on Sputnik, Viet Nam, Watergate, or John Hinckly Jr. who was found innocent by reason of insanity of attempting to assassinate the President. Murderers go free. Illegal drug sales can't be stopped. Why in hell should a teacher worry a whole lot about fraternizing with a student now and then?''

Jerry Fuller became a high school principal in 1971, and in the six years that followed there were sixteen serious sex-in-the-schools' problems he had to handle and resolve. To name a few: a custodian who liked to 'flash' (expose himself) to girls he lured into the boiler room; a homosexual teacher who seduced a student, perhaps several; an alleged gang rape that a girl invented to get attention (and she did . . . including a lot of bad publicity for Jerry and his school until she finally admitted the story was a hoax); several teachers dating their students; a coach who seduced girls regularly — he said he only had intercourse with girls who requested that he be the one to help them lose their virginity . . . and sold cocaine to students to supplement his income; a former student who asked for help because the financial aid officer at the local college wanted sexual favors in exchange for a scholarship; incest on the part of a teacher with his daughter.

''It's gotten to me, I admit,'' Fuller said. ''I still love education and being a principal, but you're asking me about sex in the schools and my experiences in dealing with it and whether or not it's on the increase. Well, the whole thing just triggers a lot of pessimism. Yes, I'd say it *is* an increasing problem. At any rate it has been in my experience. I think our country's divorce rate, which is scandalous, is another contributing factor. Kids in a single-parent family seem to have more problems and they need more attention. Therefore, they are more prone, more vulnerable to a pedophile or sex abuser.

"Then there are the models we set for both kids and teachers. I don't mean just television and X-rated movies and porno magazines, either. I know a superintendent in a district not too far away who has gone through three mistresses — all teachers in his school system — in seven years. Yes, he's married. The point is, if *I* know about him and his sex capers, you can bet a lot of people in his community know about it too. But nothing happens. A new morality? I don't know.

"What does that say to a young male teacher who is being flirted with by a high school honey whose divorced mother is seldom at home?"

* * *

That's the conclusion of the roller coaster ride.

According to Jerry Fuller, a principal now in his sixteenth year of administration, the growth and development of sex in the schools is definitely on the increase, and — somewhat paradoxically — at a time when the number of students in America's public schools is on the decline.

Based on the information obtained in the process of research for this book, we'd have to agree. The problem, though, is proving it. That is a task that is almost as impossible as presenting the causes for the illness. Any attempt to do either leads one straight down a cold, dark mine shaft.

Therefore, speculate with us that the problem *is* on the increase, and that it *does* have the potential to be as destructive to education as were declining test scores in the last decade.

Speculate, too, that it is a problem for which there are solutions, and then make a commitment to help implement those solutions.

Any nation must have a great education system to survive, to persevere. America's schools have gone through tough times and faced serious problems before, as they are now, once again. The increased incidence of sex in the schools is one of those problems — rooted in the changing moral values of our nation's people, yes, but a problem nonetheless — that must be met head on. We need only look at what the alleged sex and drug scandals in Congress in 1982 did to public confidence and good will to determine the degree to which education will be undermined if we cannot put our house in order.

Speculate in regard to the reaction of radically conservative groups — who never have supported public education and never will — such as the Moral Majority, the Ku Klux Klan and others of that ilk, if educators allow the public schools to become a modern-day reincarnation of Sodom and Gomorrah.

Do we over-dramatize the problem and its dimensions? We hope not, and we think not.

As final food for thought, please consider — hum the words in your mind — the lyrics of the song "True Love" as sung by Bing Crosby to Grace Kelly some twenty-odd years ago: ". . . and I give to you/ as you give to me/ True love/ True love . . ."

Then sing the great Elvis Presley hit "Love Me Tender" to yourself (or the recent release of the same song by Linda Ronstadt if you want to be more up to date). Beautiful lyrics, aren't they? Nice sentiment; very moral.

Now contrast them to a couple of recent hits on the Top Forty list . . . like singer Olivia Newton-John's "Let's Get Physical," and finally this one by a rock group called the Police:

"DON'T STAND SO CLOSE TO ME"

I.   *Young teacher, the subject of school-girl fantasy.*
She wants him so badly. Knows what she wants to be.
Inside her, there's longing. This girl's an open page.
Bookmarking, she's so close now. This girl is half his age.

Don't stand,
Don't stand so . . .
Don't stand so close to me.

Don't stand,
Don't stand so . . .
Don't stand so close to me.

II. *Her friends are so jealous. You know how bad girls get.*

Sometimes it's not so easy to be the teacher's pet.
Temptation. Frustration. So bad it makes him cry.
Wet bus stop, she's waiting.
His car is warm and dry.

> *Don't stand,*
> *Don't stand so . . .*
> *Don't stand so close to me.*

> *Don't stand,*
> *Don't stand so . . .*
> *Don't stand so close to me.*

III. Loose talk in the classroom. To hurt, they try and try.
Strong words in the staff room. The accusations fly.
It's no use. He sees her. He starts to shake and cough.
Just like the old man in that book by Nabokov.

> *Don't stand,*
> *Don't stand so . . .*
> *Don't stand so close to me.*

> *Don't stand,*
> *Don't stand so . . .*
> *Please don't stand so close to me.*

(Sting . . . Virgin Music Inc./Chappel Music Co. . . .
A.S.C.A.P. ©1980 A&M Records, Inc.)

Recorded by "The Police" Rock Group.

The contrast is obvious, and the ramifications are pretty clear too. Popular music, as well as movies, has always been a good barometer for educators to heed. ''How Much Is That Doggie in the Window,'' and ''Little Darlin' '' by the Diamonds, are songs that reflect a compatability with the moral code of the Fifties, just as the Beatles' ''Lucy in the Sky with Diamonds'' said a lot about youth and drugs and values in the Sixties.

If one had any doubts before, the song ''Don't Stand So Close to Me'' ought to convince them that our youth have taken the problem out of the closet and gone so far as to popularize what's going on in their music.

It's time we recognized the problem and the size of it and get to work expunging it.

Chapter 2

The Broken Taboo

A major problem for conscientious administrators who have to act upon the discovery of a sexual problem in the school is assessing the severity of a particular problem. Do you treat a faculty room innuendo as seriously as you treat the complaint of an outraged parent?

You have to ask yourself immediately, *Is this something that I wish to pursue? What will happen if I don't?* As you consider the cases and situations about to be described, keep this in mind: *What will happen if nothing is done? Is a law being broken? Is a student being harmed? Is the school system being hurt?*

If you can answer *Yes* to any of these questions, you must act, and you must act quickly.

Once you decide to act, you need guidelines for your action.

The points that follow apply to situations where teachers or other adults in the educational setting cross the line of propriety — or are accused of doing so — and become sexually involved with students.

It is dramatic to compare the steps that must be considered in dealing with a problem of sex in the schools to those that apply in solving a homicide, but the elements that need to be present once you decide to act are quite uniquely similar.

According to Lee P. Brown, Atlanta (Ga.) public safety commissioner, the man assigned the responsibility of finding the killer of Atlanta's children, at least one of these three elements is needed to solve a murder: a confession, a witness, or strong physical evidence. Two additional factors need to be considered when dealing with a problem of sex in the school, and both relate to the elements critical to solving a murder. One is the age of the student; the other is the involvement of an adult. The adult must act as an advocate for the child, whether a witness to the incident or not.

9

In proceeding to act upon such a problem, then, consider the following factors:

1. A confession of the person responsible;

2. An eyewitness;

3. Physical evidence that logically leads to the person responsible;

4. The age of the child;

5. The involvement of an adult advocate.

Look at these critical factors as you go along investigating a complaint about a teacher 'in love' or a teacher taking liberties with a student.

But *how* do you act? What exactly do you do?

Frankly, that depends. No easy steps can be recommended. There is no guarantee that if one follows certain procedures all will turn out well. However, by examining a few actual cases, it will be possible to establish how to *apply* the guidelines.

The situations that follow really happened. They have been altered only as needed to protect the innocent and the guilty.

Along the Rocky Mountain Front Range

This first example seems like a clear-cut case: if the teacher doesn't go straight to jail, he should at least lose his job and his credential. However, things don't work that simply and cleanly, as most administrators know.

According to Bill Tate, a junior high school principal in Colorado, Laurie Keables was more physically attractive than usual for a girl not quite fifteen.

"Laurie's features seemed a little harsh to me," Tate said. "Maybe it was because she pinched her lips in a pencil-thin line when she sat there, and she used too much eye-shadow and make-up. But her copper-red hair softened the toughness a little, and there was no question about it, she had a beautiful, precocious body and she dressed to show it off."

Most junior high schools have girls like Laurie Keables, those who generate lust in the hearts of men, and Laurie did just that — in the heart of an English teacher.

"Laurie came to my office and I'll never forget it," said Tate. "It was tough for both of us. The conference — if that's what you can call it — was so Laurie could tell me that not only was she maybe pregnant, but the father was Ollie Lynch. She told me that she was regularly having sex with one of my English teachers."

Tate had never been confronted with a problem like this, and for a while he came close to panic.

"They don't teach you about this sort of thing in administrative seminars. The adrenalin really flowed, but I had to stay calm and ask the right questions."

Tate asked Laurie if she had said anything to her parents about her relationship with Lynch.

"She had told no one. Just me. The more I questioned her, the more comfortable it was, strange as that sounds, and the more believable. I was amazed at how quickly something so bizarre became sort of commonplace. Laurie said that Lynch loved her and she loved him, but she was scared, especially of being pregnant. Mr. Lynch, she said, was giving her all the answers to his tests, and A's on her papers. Sort of a favor in return for her favors, I guess. Now she was afraid of what he'd do if she was going to have a baby."

Once Tate had Laurie's entire story, he decided his best course of action was to investigate as much as he could before informing her parents or confronting Lynch, the teacher.

Notice that so far, Tate only has Laurie's story, as real as it seems. He has no witnesses, no evidence, no adult advocate, and half a confession from a fourteen-year-old girl.

Tate went to Lynch's classroom and asked to see the grade book. He examined Lynch's test file, too. What Laurie had said was true: she was a straight-A student in Lynch's English class in spite of the fact that her grades in previous years had been consistent C's, and her standardized test profile in language arts and spelling was just barely average.

Tate found a test paper — completion questions — that had been made out in pencil and then erased. The paper had Laurie's name on it, but the handwriting appeared to be Lynch's.

"The test paper convinced me for certain," Tate said. "And that afternoon I confronted Ollie Lynch with the allegation. He was a young, married fellow, maybe about thirty, and turning a little soft, a little fat. If I had any doubts about Laurie's story, it was only that I found it hard to imagine what charm a guy like him would have in the eyes of a fourteen-year-old.

"According to Lynch, there was nothing happening. He denied everything, and I have to admit he was pretty convincing, in spite of my inclination not to believe him."

" 'Mr. Tate,' he said to me, 'you have to believe I'd never do that. Why, it would mean my *career*. It would destroy my marriage . . . I'd never do anything with a student. I *didn't* . . .'

"So there I was," Tate went on. "I told Mrs. Keables about her daughter's accusation and Lynch's denial. At first she said she'd file a complaint and go all the way with it. She was pretty shocked and *very* angry."

But two days later, after Bill Tate had consulted with the superintendent and the legal counsel for the district, and built his evidence file for the hearing, the roof caved in. Mrs. Keables, after a good deal of soul-searching, decided not to lodge a formal complaint against Lynch.

"She did not want to subject Laurie to the trauma of testifying, the embarrassment," Tate said. "She told me it would be too degrading, and Lynch would try to smear Laurie's character and reputation. I could see her point, but I was disappointed. I didn't know what to do."

Tate had a definite problem. In terms of the critical elements needed to handle Laurie Keables' complaint, he had next to nothing.

There was no confession from the teacher — just the opposite.

There was no eyewitness other than Laurie — a minor.

The physical evidence that might logically lead to the person responsible was flimsy, circumstantial at best, and too easy to explain away. (Lynch had told Tate that he had given Laurie an oral test and that's why the answers were in his handwriting. Laurie said it wasn't true, so it was his word against hers.)

And now there was no adult advocate for Laurie other than Tate himself.

It is possible to find a teacher or other individual guilty of making sexual advances without an adult advocate, but it's rare and it generally happens only when the student is older — usually in high school — but the point needs to be made clearly: there are no fool-proof guidelines that will apply in each and every case.

Tate might have moved to have Lynch dismissed, even

though his only witness was fourteen-year-old Laurie. It has been done. A Pennsylvania court upheld the dismissal of a teacher accused of kissing and fondling a girl in his class, even though the only witness against him was the girl herself, and her credibility was questioned. (*Wissahickon School District v. McKown*, 400 A.2d 899 (1979).

But Mrs. Keables didn't want Laurie on the witness stand.

As far as Tate was concerned, the case did not end satisfactorily. He transferred Laurie to another teacher — happily, it turned out Laurie was not pregnant — and wrote a memo for the file directing Lynch never to place himself in a one-to-one relationship with a student or he would be considered insubordinate.

As he saw it, Tate lost the case. However, in terms of the critical elements needed to determine guilt or innocence, there was nothing more he could do.

Many adults would ask why Tate and Mrs. Keables did not pursue the matter in court. Lynch's offense was, after all, the allegation of sexual assault. Tate didn't go any further for the reasons noted — he felt he lacked a case — and Mrs. Keables feared for her daughter and the impact the proceedings would have on her. Tate did, however, keep extensive documentation of the case in the event that something similar should arise later involving Lynch. Lynch, likewise, would know he was being watched. That's small comfort, but, considering the circumstances, it was the best Tate could come up with. And there was the chance that Lynch was innocent.

However, another case — perhaps more dramatic — is seen in the deep South. It illustrates what can happen if the matter of illicit sex in the schools *is* brought to trial.

Somewhere in the Deep South

The headline read "Woman Charged with Rape." According to the 1981 Associated Press story, Angela White was accused by the parents of a fifteen-year-old boy, Tom — a former student — of having given the boy drugs, alcohol, and engaging in oral sex and sexual intercourse over a two-year period.

The parents alleged they could document nearly sixty encounters from 1979 to 1981 where Ms. White, a junior high school teacher, enticed their son Tom to her apartment, gave him alcohol and marijuana, and had sex with him. Confronted with the charges of rape, sexual battery, and furnishing alcohol to a minor, Ms. White obtained an attorney and surrendered to the police.

Ms. White's lawyer maintained that she was innocent, and stated he planned a vigorous defense.

Was she guilty? At the time of this writing, the case had not yet gone to trial, but regardless of innocence or guilt, considerable damage had been suffered by both parties already. Ms. White and her husband divorced; she was asked to resign her teaching position; Tom was subjected to considerable harrassment by his peers and by the adults in his life, and transferred to another school.

Here, we don't have a confession; in fact, we have another denial from the teacher. But we certainly have an adult who is pressing for a decision in favor of the student, and we have a young man, fifteen years old, certainly too young to be anyone's lover. This is essentially the same situation as Laurie Keables' but this time with outraged parents. The administrators did act, but they have found themselves in the headlines and in the courts when they want to spend their time on the matters at hand: education.

Here is a clear example of what happens when people think they are doing the right thing, and when it appears that every choice is a bad one.

While Tom's case and Laurie Keables' are similar, the decision of Tom's parents to file the charges represents the significant difference.

One must consider, however, the wisdom of each; Tom's teacher eventually may be brought to justice for her alleged sexual harrassment of a minor because Tom's parents filed charges, but the attendant sensational publicity left its scars; Laurie's alleged seducer may have gone free, but her scars — undoubtedly just as real as Tom's — are private.

Just Over the Canadian Border

Another unique set of circumstances exists relative to the critical factors — the age of the student, the involvement of an adult, a confession, physical evidence, or a witness — and that is the possibility that the relationship between a teacher and a minor student cannot be halted.

A 1981 court case in Vancouver, British Columbia, illustrates this situation.

The parents of a fifteen-year-old boy, convinced that their son was the victim of a physical education teacher, a woman, who used sexual favors and promises of material goods to entice him to continue a relationship they considered harmful, filed charges against the teacher. They asked the court to forbid the teacher, who was in her mid-twenties, from seeing their son.

The teacher and the boy had been living together, and both agreed to submit to one-month psychological evaluations. The teacher, while denying the charges of impropriety, wanted the boy to stay with her because he had quarreled with his parents and moved out of the house. The charges of sexual favors, the teacher argued, were no more than gossip, rumor and innuendo.

The court ruled that the teacher and her fifteen-year-old student friend could continue living together until the psychological report was concluded.

As the judge put it: "Where there are allegations of sexual promiscuity . . . they are not framed as statements of fact but rather expression of opinion."

The teacher's attorney agreed. "If the assessment says the relationship is doing the boy damage, then I can't imagine the parents would take that lying down. But if it (the assessment) comes back saying 'this is a remarkable boy and he can handle it,' then you have to think you're dead in the water."

In other words, the attorney argues that while the age of the child is a factor, and there is an adult to file a complaint, still there exists no confession, no witness, and no physical or psychological evidence of harm to the child.

One begins to understand why it is important to know the five elements critical to dealing with a problem of sex in the schools, and why it is virtually impossible to provide a step-by-step process for applying the guidelines.

In the three cases presented, there were victims, but it is not always possible to determine who indeed was the prey. With Laurie Keables it may never be known. Her mother refused to be her advocate and press charges. However, with Tom and Angela White, and in the case of the Canadian boy and his P.E. teacher, there were advocates, and it must be presumed that the courts will eventually determine the true victims and the real aggressors, if any.

But Laurie Keables exemplifies one of the aggravating problems of trying to resolve a sex-in-the-schools allegation: too often it is hushed up and truth is hidden forever.

However, formal charges bring on reporters and lurid stories with banner headlines; it is usually difficult to find truth in the center of controversy and sensationalism.

It is clear that responsible adults dealing with allegations of sexual misconduct involving a child must consider the basic factors before proceeding: is there a confession; is there a witness; is there physical evidence; is the child of legal age or of exceptional maturity; is there an adult advocate?

Then the responsible person must act. The allegation must be thoroughly investigated, and it's best to seek legal advice at the outset.

A word of caution is in order. If, after investigating a charge that someone has taken a bite of the forbidden apple, guilt is determined, it is advisable to stick with the facts and stay out of the morality question. For example, had Principal Tate decided to seek the dismissal of English teacher Lynch, he would have been well-advised to charge him with statuatory rape — based on Laurie Keables' testimony — and not 'immoral conduct' or 'immorality.' Dismissal of a teacher who makes sexual advances to minor students is rarely in doubt, but 'immoral' too often touches off hopeless legal disputes, because immorality changes with the times.

Finally, it is very important to understand that most educators confronted with an allegation of sexual abuse are inclined to react much the same as Principal Tate: panic. Should the matter be pursued? What happens if it isn't? The answer is an emphatic *yes*; there must be action. To do nothing is to abrogate responsibility and invite career disaster. As Judge Marilyn Martin of Colorado Springs (Colo.) stated in a 1982 decision, after finding an elementary school principal guilty of failure to report suspicions and complaints from parents of alleged sexual assault involving a teacher and third-grade girls: "The principal owes some loyalty to his teachers — especially when he believes the allegations to be false — but he owes a higher duty to the children." The principal, it was concluded, had reasonable cause to suspect there might be child abuse, failed to report it, and was given the maximum fine for not meeting his obligation.

The message is clear. Administrators may argue strenuously that they have not been educated to handle difficult matters like sex in the school, but there is no choice. Act they must. At the very least, they must report the allegations and request investigative assistance.

Chapter 3

Teachers and Mature Students

Teen-age romances are always news and have been so since long before Shakespeare penned *Romeo and Juliet*.

Unfortunately, for many in school administration, teen love affairs are not always student-to-student. A very common problem is the young adult student who becomes entangled with a member of the faculty, as outlined in the preceeding chapter.

The guidelines presented earlier are applicable to dealing with Juliets in love or in bed with a more mature Romeo — and vice versa. When the problem presents itself, it is still appropriate to run down the list: is there a confession, is there an eyewitness, what is the age of the student, is there any phsyical evidence, is there the presence of an adult advocate.

In addition, however, there are a few other guidelines — strategies, really — that are available and need to be considered.

Three cases illustrate the application of these strategies, and also demonstrate that sometimes the love is genuine, and happy endings do occur — albeit at the expense of a near-ulcer for the administrator in charge.

The Hot Tub Romance

Judy Alvarez, a pretty high school senior enrolled in a vocational-technical school photography course somewhere in the western United States, presented the principal with the accusation that she had been in love with Will Wright, the photo instructor. She and Will had engaged in sex on twenty-seven occasions over a four-month period, Judy alleged, and she had a diary to verify it. On two dates, she said, Will took her to a motel that featured hot tubs in every room, and they engaged in sex there, too.

Will Wright, a second-year teacher with a wife and young

17

child, admitted that he and Judy were close friends, but he denied that anything inappropriate ever happened. The diary, he said, had to be the invention of an infatuated teen-ager who felt rejected by him.

"Then what about the picture you gave me?" countered Judy. "You gave me your picture and wrote on it that you'd always love me and somehow we'd work out a future together."

Judy's mother stood ready to back up a complaint of statuatory rape, and the photo — a very compelling piece of physical evidence — did exist, inscription and all, and was presented to the principal.

The case against Will Wright appeared to be very strong, the inscribed photo a most damaging item, and the diary might be circumstantial or hearsay or completely invalid, but to the principal it was very genuine and convincing.

Still, Wright adamantly denied any wrong-doing.

The district decided to suspend Wright with pay pending an investigation into Judy Alvarez's charges, and turned to their legal counsel for advice. The action recommended and subsequently carried out represents one of the additional strategies available to school administrators who must determine truth in very trying situations.

The strategy: if legal in your state or city, request that the persons involved submit to a polygraph — a lie detector — test.

In Will Wright's case, the courts permitted the admission of polygraph test results as evidence, and while he refused to take the exam, Judy Alvarez was more than willing to comply. She passed with flying colors. According to the expert who administered the polygraph test, Judy Alvarez was telling the complete truth.

The district administrators concluded that the polygraph results, coupled with the rest of the evidence, constituted good cause for the termination of Will Wright.

That's exactly what they did, and although Wright appealed his dismissal, the Board of Education upheld the administration's recommendation. Wright chose not to pursue the issue any further.

The use of the polygraph test, then, to augment or verify evidence and testimony in a sex-in-schools problem, is a strategy that should be considered carefully. It must be recognized that in some states the lie detector test is not viewed as legal or appropriate evidence. Recognize, too, that care must be taken to ensure that the person administering a polygraph examination is expert and has a sound reputation. The best way to be certain requires working through the police department. There are, according to most authorities, many unreliable quacks purporting to be expert polygraph examiners.

A Proposition in the Pines

A second example, which illustrates another strategy available to administrators in cases where the five guidelines do not apply, occurred in Texas.

A high school social studies teacher in charge of an outdoor education field trip to a wilderness area in Texas — we'll call him James O'Neill — found himself in the principal's office a week after the group returned from the experience. One of the senior girls who went on the trip, eighteen-year-old Maureen Taylor, had told the principal that O'Neill kissed her often while they were in the wilds, petted her and tried to remove her blouse, and three times invited her to spend the night in his tent.

"Absolutely not true!" protested O'Neill. "I worked too hard to develop this outdoor program and trip, and to make it a success. I'd never do anything to jeopardize it or me. Maureen is lying."

Several factors influenced the principal, Art Bradley, to employ the strategy that eventually resolved the matter. First, he had no confession. Nor did he have any physical evidence or eyewitness. The age of the alleged victim was not a factor, and while Maureen's parents knew about her complaint against O'Neill, they were not inclined to press charges. Indeed, there was no real criminal charge — inappropriate behavior, perhaps sexual harrassment, maybe sexual assault. The ambiguity of the situation aggravated principal Bradley. Finally, there was O'Neill's reputation and Maureen Taylor's reputation.

"I had an allegation of sexual advances that was marginal," Bradley said. "But I also had the fact that O'Neill was known as a pot smoker and a teacher who had made some moves on students before. Then I had Maureen Taylor, a beautiful, sincere, intense young lady who was practically a straight-A student and a model in terms of conduct. No doubt in my mind at all that she was telling the truth. Hell, it broke her up to come tell me. She idolized O'Neill for getting the program off the ground. It crushed her when he tried to bed her in the woods."

The polygraph was not an option available to Bradley, but he consulted with his superintendent and got the go-ahead to use what constitutes another strategy for handling sex-in-the-schools problems: the element of bluff.

Admittedly, it's best to resort to bluff — some call it persuasion — only when critical factors are absent, but if the administrator is convinced that improper behavior has taken place, then the careful application of the bluff may be in order, and it can be effective.

Better still, it can be *quietly* effective.

Principal Bradley's remarks illustrate the application of the bluff. "I went to the boss and laid out the case. I argued that I had to do something, even though I knew I didn't have enough goods to warrant the use of our attorneys. But I had my hands full and my pants to hold up, as far as I was concerned. The outdoor education program was getting a bad reputation because of a weak and troublesome teacher, and the thought of that creep propositioning a young girl made me damned mad.

"So I asked the supe to back me up. I would tell O'Neill that the case was shaky, sure enough, but I was going to recommend him for termination. He could fight it. He might even win, and I told him so when we actually met. But by heaven O'Neill was going to have the accusation out in the public. He could resign quietly, or he could prepare to fight it."

Bradley implemented the plan and as far as he was concerned, the bluff was successful. O'Neill, still protesting his innocence, agreed to resign rather than face the dismissal recommendation and subsequent hearing.

"To tell the truth," Bradley said, "O'Neill knew as well as I did that Maureen Taylor was not lying. Let him resign with a face-saving denial, just so long as he resigns. To me, that was *prima facia* evidence that he was guilty."

Perhaps, perhaps not. It can be argued that principal Bradley's use of the bluff was unfair to O'Neill, and that O'Neill deserved help and counseling instead of firing, but the point to be made is that bluff or persuasion is a strategy administrators can add to their arsenal of tools for dealing with sex in the schools. Further, if the administration is willing to back the principal and support the recommendation to terminate, it may be a misnomer to call the action a bluff. Moreover, in Bradley's case, it removed the principal from being the sole judge and jury and let the accused know that someone else would hear and decide the truth of the matter.

Till Death Do You Part

A third strategy or guideline that needs to be noted has to do with *rumors* of sex or love relationships in schools — usually high schools, but not always. It's difficult to state this guideline succinctly. In colloquial terms, the old cliche "If the truck runs, don't fix it" gets the concept across. Perhaps a better phrasing might be: if you don't have a case, don't go to court.

There are many examples to illustrate the guideline or strategy at issue here. In general, this one comes into play in those many cases where there really is no hard data. What you do have is a persistent, nagging rumor that someone is taking liberties with a student, or the unfounded accusation that a teacher is dating or loving a student. Or, to complicate things a bit, you may have some evidence that a teacher and student are getting physical, but the student has not complained, nor has the parent. As the administrator, you have not much more than an etherial vapor, but that doesn't mean you don't have a problem. Most likely, if *you* are privy to the rumor, then so are a lot of parents and teachers, and sooner or later they will march angrily into your office and demand that something be done.

Example. A high school principal in Illinois was approached by the chairman of the math department.

"Listen," the teacher said. "I think you ought to know it's pretty common knowledge that Bill Swift (one of the school's math teachers) is romancing Melinda Callahan." In providing this bit of confidential information, the department head implied heavily that the teacher and student regularly went to bed together.

Bill Swift was young and single. The principal checked things out and discovered that Swift and Melinda were seen together often.

But what to do about it, the principal wondered. He decided, very correctly, to let Bill Swift know that rumors were circulating about Melinda and him.

"He didn't deny it," the principal said, somewhat amazed. "In fact, he said he and Melinda *were* very good friends, and he went to her home occasionally, and her parents approved of the relationship, and he assured me there would never be anything inappropriate at school. He would 'keep it cool,' so to speak."

The principal conceded that he nearly developed ulcers worrying about the potential for trouble with this romance, especially in light of the conservatism of the community. But Bill Swift kept his word; there were no problems. In June, following graduation, the principal received an engraved invitation to the wedding of Melinda Callahan and Bill Swift.

"That was more than five years ago," the principal related. "Bill still teaches here, and from all I can see, he and Melinda are truly living happily ever after."

In conducting research interviews, the above example is typical of what appears to be a fairly prevalent occurrence in America's high schools. Cases were reported from nearly every state, and while most of them were about high school students and their teachers, several were about elementary and junior high or middle school children and teachers.

Two classic cases. In Kentucky a teacher transferred to the next grade level each year for five years — beginning in the third grade — so she could have in her class a boy with whom she developed a very loving relationship, according to the superintendent. The parents of the boy, both former teachers, were aware of the 'friendship' and advised the superintendent that they were not concerned about the teacher fondling, kissing and hugging their son. "After all," they said, "none of it happens at school, so why should you be concerned if we aren't." Well, for good or no, the superintendent *is* concerned, and hopes to slow down the relationship by making certain the woman teacher does not obtain a transfer beyond the eighth-grade-level assignment.

The second case, in California: a male seventh-grade teacher fell in love with an eighth-grade girl at his school. He walked her to class holding hands, bought her gifts. The administration advised him to cease and desist; he told the administration to pound sand, to mind their own business. The administrators informed the girl's parents, who said the teacher was a fine man (even though he was married at the time). The teacher was transferred to another building. However, when the girl entered high school, the teacher divorced his wife, dated the girl through high school and college, and finally married her.

The third guideline again, then, is not to pursue a case where none exists, where there is no complaint. Monitor the situation, of course. Confront and advise the teacher of the serious consequences that can occur. Consider transferring a teacher to cool off a budding relationship that appears to be developing into something more than platonic. But recognize, too, that what is happening — a teacher falling in love with a student — can be within the bounds of legal if not appropriate conduct, and there's nothing you can do about it.

Therefore, don't.

\

Chapter 4

Homosexuality

While working in the district office, one of the authors sat in the superintendent's office and overheard the superintendent's half of a telephone conversation which went as follows:

"Yes, that's right. Um hmm. He worked in this district. Yes. Well . . . um . . . well, he resigned. That's right. For personal reasons. Mmm? His, not mine.

"What were they? Well, ah . . . I'm afraid they were personal. I really can't elaborate much more than that.

". . . Well, let's just say that he used poor judgment in his personal dealings with students. . . . Yes. And it was better that he severed relationships with the school district.

"What do I mean 'poor judgment'? Let me put it this way, he gave an eighth-grade boy a monkey bite."

That's poor judgment, no doubt about it.

When asked why he was so evasive at first with the caller, the superintendent explained. "One thing you can never be sure about is who you're talking with. That could have been the teacher's attorney trying to find out what I was telling a possible employer. To tell the truth, we never did fire the guy for sex-related offenses. As far as our records go, he was an excellent teacher. He probably was, for that matter, except for his tendency to give a monkey bite here and there. He just resigned in the middle of the year. I had the goods on him, but we never did anything once he agreed to move on.

"He had a lot of yard work around his house and he hired some of the boys in his seventh and eighth-grade classes to help him out. One of them went home with a big hickey on his neck and the kid's parents — as you might expect — wanted to know where it came from. In this town, a monkey bite is almost as newsworthy as a space ship landing in the supermarket parking lot. Anyway, when the boy told his parents that he and his

24

teacher were wrestling and the teacher gave him the bite, the parents hit the roof.

"They had the boy and two of his friends tell me the story. I believed them and I confronted the teacher with the story. He didn't deny it at all. He asked if he could resign, and the parents agreed that if he did, they'd call it a wash and not press charges. They figured their boy had suffered enough without charges and counter charges and newspaper coverage. The whole thing was kept quiet and out of the press.

"Maybe I should have pushed it, but I counselled him out. I urged him to get some help. Maybe this guy was a child molester. I don't know. I *do* know that he's not molesting children in my district anymore. And I know, too, that I have to be careful about what I tell people. I should never have said what I just said on the phone. I'm pretty sure that it wasn't a lawyer who called, but it could have been, and if it was I'd have big trouble right now."

The above case is of particular interest because it illustrates most of the major elements that surface when one deals with the problem of homosexual behavior in the schools:

1. The issue was never the teacher's private sex life, his homosexuality. The issue was what he did with young boys.

2. The teacher did not fight the accusations made by the parents and the superintendent.

3. There was no suggestion of love in the situation.

4. The parents were quick to act against the teacher and to support the superintendent.

Bear these points in mind as the examples that follow are presented; the pattern seems to be consistent with regard to them.

The Homosexual Teacher

A homosexual teacher is protected by law, common sense, and — hopefully — good administrative judgment. A person's sexual preferences outside the workplace should not constitute a reason for dismissal. Sex habits become an area of concern and investigation only when and if they come into the classroom.

Two cases where the teacher's sexual life outside school came to the attention of the administration demonstrate this point. While the first example does not deal expressly with homosexuality, it makes the point clearly.

A Sex Change in the Far West

Anne Dunlop was a girls' physical education teacher until she took an extended leave for medical reasons. The district administration was more than a little surprised when she returned to work not as Anne, but as Dan Dunlop . . . a man.

Dan's superintendent was quick to launch his argument that the role model Dunlop represented was just too much for the students in his district to handle, and he initiated proceedings to dismiss him.

The press had a field day. Dunlop was never charged with immoral acts with students; he therefore fought the charges and did so with the support of the local professional association. Dunlop argued that his previous evaluations when he was a woman were good, and that the sex change operation did nothing to impair or reduce his teaching effectiveness. In fact, he argued, it probably helped.

However, the district prevailed, and Dunlop lost his job.

The evidence presented and the arguments of the administration convinced the court that Dunlop's teaching would suffer because of student and community reaction to his operation. His notoriety was just too great for the students not to be adversely influenced. Parents, reasoned the administration, had the right to expect a more traditional role model in a teacher.

Though the district won the case, one must ponder the human cost. There is little point in arguing that having a sex change is an appropriate or inappropriate way to handle an emotional, physical or sexual problem. The merits of the drastic solution are beyond the scope of the authors' intentions here, but it *is* proper to suggest that an astute administrator should keep an eye on the classroom performance of the teacher rather than on lurid matters that have more bearing on the emotions and values of the people in charge than on the skills of the teacher being hired and fired.

There is much to recommend that Dunlop should have *not* been fired immediately on return from medical leave. The administration could have taken a wait-and-see attitude and let him teach for a reasonable period of time, evaluating him continually and carefully, of course. Dunlop may have been an excellent teacher despite the sex change. He may also have been a failure. Perhaps the strain on the faculty and the students would have been too much for all concerned; dismissal would have then been legitimate, and it would have been based on cause, not prejudice.

There is a point, of course, when a person's private sexual life *does* have bearing on the classroom, and the courts have been reasonably clear about this circumstance. For example, the courts did not support a school district's efforts to fire a woman who was rumored to be sexually involved with a man who shared her home, but the courts did support a district that fired a woman for belonging to a sex club and publicly advocating — among other things — group sex.

Clearly, judging one's sex life becomes a matter of degree, but the measurement of that degree must start at the point where harm is being done to students. This is a firm guideline to remember.

A second and less complex case will help clarify the difference between the private sexual activities of a non-heterosexual teacher, and those of a teacher who takes advantage of students regardless of sexual preference.

Perversion in Seattle Suburbia

David Sampson was a respected teacher in his district, a suburb of Seattle. He had a good record, and his evaluations were consistently positive for all of the fifteen years he taught intermediate math.

It was with great surprise that Sampson's superintendent, Ken Lawson, read in the morning paper that the teacher had been arrested for lewd and lascivious behavior with minors. Sampson, among other things, was accused of having provided beer and marijuana to minors. As soon as he finished the article, Lawson called his substitute teacher service and made certain that a sub was ready. He then notified the principal of the school that if Sampson showed up he was not to be permitted to teach; Lawson was placing him on immediate suspension. Under state law, a teacher accused of any sex crime is placed on a compulsory leave of absence.

To say that the evidence against Sampson was powerful is to

be guilty of understatement. A parent had filed the complaint against him, and when police searched his apartment they found photographs of unidentified nude boys, and they found pictures that Sampson had taken of several of his students.

Here, in a world of almost right and almost wrong, is a black and white case. Open and shut. Sampson was wrong and he had no right to continue teaching. It was clear that he took advantage of his teaching job to prey on children and satisfy his sexual appetite.

Superintendent Lawson did not hesitate as he proceeded for dismissal. The case was sound. There was a parent advocate; the boys were under age, none over fourteen; there was no confession from Sampson, but the physical evidence was compelling. The teacher association declined to offer Sampson comfort or legal support.

Sampson was terminated promptly.

Consider again the point made at the beginning of this chapter, the second element common to dealings with homosexuals: the teacher did not choose to fight the allegations or the dismissal action. The taboo against abusing children for sexual pleasure is so strong that when it is coupled with our society's general distaste for homosexuality, the teacher has little ground for legal recourse.

Dan Dunlop had good cause to argue that his sex change did not impair his teaching ability; his district, though it won the dismissal case, was on shaky ground. No laws were broken, no child was harmed.

On the other hand, David Sampson was guilty of a crime, there were victims and evidence, and there were parents who wanted him punished. As in the case of the teacher who inflicted the monkey bite, the parents were quick to seek the teacher's dismissal.

With these strong attitudes working in our society, it is no wonder that the teacher caught in an illegal situation with a youngster of the same sex — a homosexual relationship — is reluctant to try to fight dismissal proceedings.

The teacher involved in heterosexual harrassment, on the other hand, can sometimes find begrudging or tacit understanding of the indiscretions, even from the family of the victim, on occasion.

The point, then, bears repeating. Our fears and prejudices make us quick to act against homosexuals. We should always, however, regardless of the sexual combination at issue, keep our concern for the students and the harm done to them foremost in mind. We need to perceive that even though both Sampson, who seduced young boys, and Dunlop, who had a sex change, suffered the same punishment — dismissal — their situations were not at all equal.

Another case demonstrates that the teacher's private life is not the issue, while the effect on the students is, and the impact of gossip may or may not be damaging, depending on what the administrators involved do about it.

An 'AC/DC' in the Great Lakes Region

Leroy Bennett, a high school teacher in the Great Lakes region, had a spotty record. His evaluations were a series of lukewarm statements.

His principal had made some suggestions about improving his teaching, but there were never any specific charges made against Bennett, and dismissal had never been attempted. The principal had made written reference to Bennett's absenteeism, particularly on Mondays and Fridays. The principal, James DeRieux, usually relied on hall gossip, informal conversations with students, and phone calls from parents for his source of evaluative information.

It needs to be noted that if gossip about a teacher is good, the evaluation is perfunctory. Conversely, if student and parent gossip is negative and complaining, the teacher is scrutinized more carefully, though often the formal evaluation that results is not specific in regard to weaknesses.

Such was Bennett's case. Criticism was vague, almost misty, and never specific. Couple this with the fact that no teachers had been fired by the district where Bennett worked — at least not to the memory of the eldest staff members. The worst that had happened to Bennett was a short reminder that was not documented about 'problems.' As DeRieux put it: "I think it's better to handle these kinds of negative things lightly, so I keep the system moving efficiently. Most teachers are really pretty good and it doesn't help anyone if I'm on their back all the time."

Most students liked Bennett. They enjoyed his sarcastic sense of humor, his facetious remarks, and his 'sense of style.' If Pontiac produced a new hot model car, for example, Bennett bought one. He could talk with authority about sports cars and racing.

Most believed that he had at one time raced sports cars at tracks in the Midwest.

A bachelor, twice-divorced, Bennett displayed an air of independence, a lack of concern for the school system's rules that endeared him to some. He was considered handsome in a clean-cut though somewhat jaded-faded way, one fellow teacher commented. His peers liked to tease him often about his hangovers.

Bennett's marriages had failed, but only his second wife and a few close friends knew that he occasionally disappeared on weekends to Detroit to cruise as a gay prostitute. His first wife finally left him when she could no longer tolerate his unexplained though subtly understood disappearances, which he later referred to as 'lust weekends.'

He had a series of more intense affairs with various gay businessmen in the Detroit area, but none lasted more than six months. During his second marriage, he managed to balance his family and his gay affairs, but the tension finally caused an explosion. Both of his wives explained that they could almost tolerate his deviancy from the marital norm because he was such a charming, intelligent and exciting husband.

After his second wife left him, alone in his apartment one evening, a student from school came to call — knocking wildly at the door. Bennett, who privately admitted that he was a little drunk at the time, opened the door and let the young man from one of his social studies classes enter.

The boy came in as if pursued by demons, and had it been a movie scene, Bennett commented, the special effects would have included thunder and lightning.

"Mr. Bennett," the boy cried out, "you've got to help me. I'm as queer as a son of a bitch and someone's got to help me understand it."

Sober enough to keep his eyes focused on his steady pay check, Bennett responded. "I'll help any of my students, but why do you think I can do you any good in this situation?"

"My god, Mr. Bennett, you're gay just like me and I know that you understand."

Maybe he could be chided by some of his homophile brothers, maybe it was a breach of personal ethic, maybe it was the better part of valor or discretion. Whatever it was, Bennett only hesitated a moment before he said, "I can sympathize with you for sure, but what makes you think I'm gay like you think you are?"

"Come on, Mr. Bennett. I *know*. Everyone else suspects you are, but I *know*. I can tell."

"Well, *if* I was gay, I'd deny it. And besides, I'm not. Now, tell me what's bothering you."

The boy went on to tell his tale of sexual doubt and unhappiness, including what would happen if his father found out about his fears. Bennett listened carefully and sympathetically, never making a comment that could be interpreted as encouragement.

He sent the boy home with the usual advice — fairly sound in spite of its triteness — that you are who you are and that people have many ways of satisfying themselves, and homosexuality isn't necessarily bad.

Bennett said later that he wished he had been more supportive to and honest with the young man, but he felt that any effort to support the boy's homosexuality would have done him in at the district office with people who were already barking at his heels enough about his absenteeism and drinking. He couldn't afford to have it rumored that he was in his own apartment alone with a boy who was telling people he was gay.

The district office, in spite of their various concerns about Bennett, never went for dismissal on the grounds of homosexuality. As the vice-principal who handled some of the evaluations said, "We'd have been crazy to try. His private life didn't affect his teaching. As far as we know, he never took advantage of a student. We did make a half-hearted attempt to get him for drinking and excessive absences because that *did* influence his teaching effectiveness. He would sometimes come to work reeking of gin and we'd talk to him about it. Sure, there were rumors of his being gay, but we never thought it was a problem we could move on."

On analysis, this seems to be a logical way to proceed in terms of Bennett's homosexuality. The problem was not that Bennett wasn't fired for being a homosexual, it was more that the administration didn't fire him for other cause, and did a poor job of evaluation. Bennett's erring ways — missing many Mondays and Fridays, coming to work smelling of alcohol, and poor preparation — should have been carefully and systematically documented, and he should have been given the opportunity to correct the problems. Failing to improve, he should have been fired.

Bennett's case was much different from that of Gary Reimer, a driver education teacher in Florida. Reimer was caught by the police performing oral sex with a seventeen-year-old hitchhiker, not one of his students.

Reimer was dismissed immediately, and rightly so. The case was very clear, like that of Lawson who was arrested and who had nude photographs of some of his students. Reimer could reasonably be expected to take advantage of his own students in driver ed cars. If he was driven by his desires enough to risk committing a sex act in a parked car, he could be expected to take similar risks with students. Again, as is so often the case, Reimer did not contest the district's action. Again, as happens frequently in homosexual problems, the teacher association declined to become involved and offer assistance.

Is It Love or Is It Lust?

There is the problem of lust and love to consider. In the list of elements at the beginning of this chapter, it is stated that homosexual problems in the school do not appear to involve love. This is a phenomenon that goes beyond the scope of this book and its intent.

To say that the problems with homosexual teachers usually do not involve a teacher falling in love with a student is not to say that homosexuals do not fall in love or that heterosexuals have the corner on the love market.

What has been observed, rather, is that when a problem of a homosexual teacher surfaces, the specific incident is usually what is classified as a casual act. Most of the incidents subjected to interviews for this book seemed to involve fleeting passion, acts of compulsion.

In the cases researched, problems of homosexuality seemed to involve hidden photographs, parked cars, furtive embraces, police. It is suspected that this is due more to our society's values than to the long-range interests of homosexuals. Our society is more tolerant of heterosexual affairs and is more shocked and far less sophisticated or objective about homosexual affairs. Therefore, only the most blatant examples surface.

It appears that there is some degree of private sympathy for the male or female teacher who is attracted to a younger person of the opposite sex; apparently we can allow ourselves to be a little more understanding. But with the homosexual, our fears and prejudices make the encounters furtive and seamy.

In none of the interviews was there a case where a teacher

was trying to establish a long-term relationship or affair with a student of the same sex. This, of course, makes it easier for an administrator to deal with the problem, to put it bluntly.

Once again, a wise administrator should spend a moment reflecting — is it the teacher's role with students or the administrator's prejudices that become the basis for whatever action is taken?

To summarize, the guidelines that emerge for consideration when one is confronted with the problem of a homosexual teacher are first to determine whether or not the individual's sexual preferences interfere with students' learning. If it isn't possible to prove a connection, it's best to forget about it, regardless of your personal attitudes regarding 'gays.' Second, it is generally true that a teacher's private life has no bearing on his or her effectiveness in the classroom, but there are exceptions, as noted in the two cases cited where students and other children were seduced and photographed by the offenders.

Third, concern for the students and the harm that may become them must be kept foremost in mind.

Finally, recognize that most Americans fear and harbor prejudice for the homosexual. In investigating an allegation of sex in the schools that involves homosexual behavior, be diligent in maintaining an objective — not an angry or emotional — attitude.

Chapter 5

Love and Lust in the Faculty Lounge

"I've always said I was one woman who could never be raped . . ."

The quote is from an elementary teacher, Sharon King, and the interview detailing how she *was* raped — by a fellow teacher — is related in this chapter.

It's interesting. If you approach educators, be they teachers, principals, counselors or central office administrators, about the problem of teacher-to-teacher romances or sexual encounters, you'll likely get one of two responses: one, it does not happen here and it never will; two, there have been some romances among employees that budded here, but the people were both unattached and it was a beautiful romance that ended in an idyllic marriage.

If you approach people in the business world, the response to the question about employee romance is likely to be far more honest.

There are lots of school districts where the two responses stated above represent the state of affairs accurately; however, there are a few additional degrees of entanglement that constitute reality, and they range from sexual harrassment to date rape* and sexual attack. Definitely, they are not pretty, not idyllic, and not liaisons of benefit to anyone concerned, and they do happen in most school systems regularly.

Sexual harrassment is dealt with in a later chapter, although at least one incident described here falls into that category and serves to illustrate a point about love and lust among faculty members.

---

*The term 'date rape' is defined by most experts as a sex activity between two people that is beyond what one party, usually the woman, considers acceptable. It's the "if you really love me you'll do it" sexual involvement; it can be petting, it can be the sex act.

A young, unmarried high school principal named Jerry Lehman commenced a year-long romance with a guidance counselor on his staff, Sally McAllister. The relationship began to falter during the summer, however, and there were rumors about lovers' spats becoming more and more frequent.

"I'm tired of it," Sally confided to friends. "I've tried to break up, to tell Jerry it's over, but he won't give in. He's harrassing me."

Sally arrived at work one morning in September with a broken headlight on her car, and said Lehman had smashed it in anger when she refused to allow him to enter her apartment that weekend. "It's over, I keep telling him, but he won't go away. He won't accept it. I'm scared."

As the new school year settled into a comfortable routine, Sally McAllister filed harrassment and destruction of property charges against Jerry Lehman. Local newspaper headlines trumpeted the news: "Lehman Romance Probe Set."

Lehman, who may or may not have been guilty of harrassment — he refused to comment on the matter other than to say he had tried to talk with Sally about their relationship, but he had never followed her or tampered with her car — was now himself being harrassed, by Sally and by the press and by his superintendent, who began his own investigation of the situation.

The incident was settled quietly. Sally and Jerry, through their attorneys, reached a peaceful understanding; the romance, for certain, came to an end. The press, initially eager to print copy about a possible sex scandal at the high school, lost interest when it became evident there would be no testimony in court to follow and report. The superintendent concluded that no disciplinary action was warranted.

The point to be emphasized, however, is that the broken romance was embarrassing, if not outright damaging, to the reputations and careers of both Jerry Lehman and Sally McAllister. While most love affairs don't end with formal charges of harrassment by one party against the other, it needs to be recognized that the potential for that eventuality is always present. The publicity that results is particularly bad for educators. A bank executive might romance one of his tellers and end up in the newspapers just as Lehman did, but the public's tolerance is much greater for erring businessmen than it is when the person being grieved is an educator, particularly a school principal.

That's the first major guideline educators need to understand in regard to office romances: stepping into a faculty affair is often as potentially dangerous as stepping into quicksand. Eyebrows raise. Gossip flows, and if things go sour, the 'Ain't That Awful' syndrome can become an ugly roar.

What to do about it? One can't pass a board policy prohibiting faculty members from dating and falling in love. One can, however, offer the parties some advice: Be careful. The fish bowl wherein educators spend their careers is very public, and the moral values applied to the behavior of teachers and educators are far more rigid than for others. In the public's eye, it's no longer a cardinal sin for educators to drink and smoke, but the standards for romantic and sexual behavior remain Reagan-rigid. *Playboy* and *Penthouse* are no-nos for teachers, most parents will agree, and it's strictly bad form for principals to kick out the headlights of their girl friends' cars, especially when the lady in question is a faculty member.

An annual talk with the faculty about community standards and expectations for educators is not an absurd suggestion. Teachers and administrators, particularly young and inexperienced folks, might titter a bit at such a 'sermon,' but a few well-chosen examples should raise their level of concern and lower the giggles as effectively as reviews of lawsuits against teachers for acts of negligence tend to command serious attention and sober reflections.

While considering the advisability of a fireside chat with employees about the inherent dangers of love in the faculty lounge, examine some additional examples.

* * *

Dan Gillespie, an administrator with an exemplary record of accomplishments, found himself in a romantic complication that provided a new dimension to the term 'mid-life crisis,' and contained all the elements necessary for a good novel. Gillespie's dilemma, however, was all too real.

"I was at a weekend workshop I'd helped design," Dan said. "We were into improving teacher performance and generating teacher renewal through the use of school climate improvement techniques. We held the workshops in a private lodge, an old Y camp, located an hour's drive from town in a beautifully forested spot. We did that on purpose. We wanted the teachers to totally immerse themselves in the activities with nothing to distract them. We conducted the sessions, ate our meals, and slept in the same large motel-like lodge.

"We had already conducted two workshops the first year with great results and no problems," said Gillespie, "so I was more or less blind-sided, hit by lightning, when it happened.

"It was late the second evening, after the wrap-up. We were all going home the next morning, and when the group broke up a bunch of people decided to go for a late-night walk through the woods. It was cold, misty, almost foggy-white out, and the forest was beautiful that night. We all felt a warm glow, both from the good feelings the workshop had created and the wine we drank together after the final session.

"I was enjoying the walk and the cold air. I was moving right along at a fast pace to catch up with the group. Then out of the mist I saw one of the teachers — Jenny — coming toward me, back toward the lodge.

" 'Too cold?' I asked her. And then I was flabbergasted. She said no, she was looking for me, and she wrapped herself around me and began kissing me.

"Jenny was a good ten years younger than me, divorced, a damned good-looking woman, and I couldn't believe what was happening."

What was happening, said Dan Gillespie, was the beginning of an extramarital romance that he knew was potential disaster, and he wrestled with his conscience — he loved his wife and family — and his flattered ego. The battle went on for nearly six months before Gillespie was able to resolve the matter.

"Jenny didn't want to hurt me," he said. "She just loved me, she said. I guess I represented the security she wanted and needed in her life and she found me attractive. Hell, I was just dumb flattered and infatuated. She didn't intend any sexual harrassment, like to get a better job or some special treatment because of my position. Nevertheless, I *was* harrassed as hell over the thing, I can tell you."

After six months Dan Gillespie reached his decision. "It helped that we'd never gone the full route," he said. "You can believe that or not, but in a way that was what helped me decide it had to end. I'd been seeing Jenny, dropping over to her apartment for a drink after a meeting, or sometimes instead of a meeting, and we'd talk, sometimes neck like a couple of teen-age kids. I liked her. I was flattered by her love, her admiration for me, my jokes, my whatever-it-was that attracted her to me. But we did not make love. We never went to bed. And then I realized that it didn't make any difference. We might just as well have, because if anyone found out we were seeing each other like this they would never believe we hadn't.

"So that's when I told Jenny, 'no more of this.' She cried. She said we could be lovers and she wouldn't push me to marry, but I guess I knew that would never work. Thank god she did not retaliate or threaten. It just ended. Clean. Sad, yes. But in the long run I think it salvaged her career, not to mention mine and my marriage, and we're both just better off in the long haul. I think even she sees that now.

"You know," Gillespie concluded, "I didn't really love Jenny. It was just an adolescent fantasy that almost came true when I was in my forties. It was hell. Jenny was beautiful. She *is* a beautiful woman. It showed me, though, how these things happen, and how easy it is to step across that line and become involved in something you know is wrong. I understand a little better how so many guys my age end up divorced and messed up."

Dan Gillespie was fortunate, as he saw it. His point about sexual involvement is valid, and it is a lesson to be underscored. Whether or not Jenny and Dan went to bed and had sex during the course of their 'romance' is irrelevant. If the affair had been made public, it would be presumed by most people that they had been physically intimate.

* * *

Going back to the frequently stated response to the question about love in the faculty lounge — "it doesn't happen here and it never will" — one begins to question the honesty and integrity of those who make such head-in-the-sand pronouncements.

In point of fact, if education is comparable to the business world, and if Patrice and Jack Horn are right about what they say in their book *Sex in the Office* — that there is at least one Romeo and one office vamp in every organization — then it's probably safer to accept the conclusions offered earlier by principal Jerry Fuller: it *does* exist and it's on the increase.

The occurrences cited so far in this chapter represent an extremely small sample, admittedly. However, in conducting research, it became very clear that the most frequently volunteered cases were those about faculty members getting intimate — or being so accused, at any rate — with other faculty members.

Let's verify that. The following letter, sent to the writers from a Midwestern city, came in response to an ad in a national journal seeking information about the problem. It speaks for itself:

To Whom It May Concern:

This incident did not happen to me, but I have watched a dear friend destroy her career in a neighboring suburban school district by falling in love with her principal.

She was married for only ten months when her husband ran off with a neighbor, leaving her (let's call her Ann) and had some terrific teaching projects going. He was a great guy, married with three children. I was divorced. Nothing ever came of my love for him. In fact, I doubt that he ever knew how very much I cared for him.

At the same school, one of the male teachers who was divorced began dating a female teacher, a widow, and their romance was common knowledge. They finally married, but it did not work out. What it did cause was a lot of marital spats, often main events, that spilled over into the halls at school and disrupted things a lot.

The fourth case I know about involved a white, male principal, married with two children, who stepped out with one of his black teachers, who was also married. The affair became so bold that the two of them began disappearing over the noon hour, and she often left her class unattended. The administration heard about it and finally transferred the principal to another school. He never admitted to having an affair, and there hasn't been a breath of scandal since he was moved. The matter was never officially investigated.

I hope these true stories will help you in your research.

Sincerely,

NAME WITHHELD

The authenticity of the four cases described by the teacher who wrote the letter may be questioned, because we have chosen not to pursue the leads she provided, but the fact that the educator in Missouri took time to write down the experiences and sign her real name to the letter speaks for itself. Furthermore, each instance described was that of a faculty member involved with another staff member.

Finally, before an effort is made to find some order in all the chaos that the examples presented here seem to represent, review the experience of Sharon King — mentioned at the beginning of this chapter — who volunteered to be interviewed and have her story tape recorded.

Sharon King, an elementary teacher, was raped by another teacher. She never reported the crime to the police or to school authorities, and one has to admit that her reason for not doing so has some credibility.

According to Sharon, she was reading a book in bed on a warm fall night some years back. Her husband, also a teacher, was gone on an overnight trip to nearby Chicago, and their four children were in bed sleeping.

"About 9:30 that night," related Sharon, "just out of the blue I heard the front screen door open and footsteps, and then Clyde walked into the room and sat down on the bed. He had a six-pack of beer.

"I said 'hi,' and I can't tell you how embarrassed I was. I hadn't locked the screen door, for one thing. And, I mean Clyde and his wife were friends, and we went out dancing and played cards, but we weren't accustomed to seeing one another like this. I was in my nightgown.

"I said, 'Listen, Clyde, excuse me a second and I'll get my robe and come out in the kitchen and we can talk.' He said that was okay and went to the kitchen. I was confused, but he was a friend and a fellow teacher at my school, so I joined him in the kitchen.

"Clyde opened the beer and then suggested that I put on some records, and before I knew it he was talking to me like a guy on the make. I couldn't believe it. It was sort of like if my brother was doing this to me. Just not believable.

"He began pawing me, and saying 'Come on, Sharon.' If you've ever seen something like that in a movie or on television, that's how I felt. It was like a scene out of a movie. I kept trying to get out of the situation, but Clyde was strong.

"I've always said I was one woman who could never be raped, because I'm pretty strong myself, but I could not get out of his grip. I fought him . . . a long time . . . but I have no recollection of how long. I thought I could wear him down, and I didn't want to scream and wake up the kids.

"Finally, after I don't know how long, he pinned me to the couch and was able to penetrate. I was just . . . I mean I felt like I was tainted. Absolutely dirty. I had let it happen.

"When he was finished, he let me up and I locked myself in the bathroom until I heard him leave."

Why didn't Sharon King report Clyde? Why didn't she file a criminal complaint?

"I was afraid my husband would kill him, or blame me. I was afraid his reaction would be violent — against me or Clyde, or both."

Can any sense come from the varied examples of love and lust on faculty row presented here? Are there any guidelines or rules to be gleaned from a more careful examination of the data?

It seems clear that the first point, already mentioned, is to recognize the need to articulate the dangers of faculty liaisons and romances. For that matter, the danger to one's career, the danger of becoming a victim like Sharon King, exists in *any* work place. Therefore, administrators should *talk* about the problem with their staff: Heighten awareness of all employees about the harm that can come their way; make certain no one is taking the attitude that 'it can't happen to me.' Both Dan Gillespie and Sharon King will testify that it *can* happen and it *does* happen to people who least expect to be faced with an uninvited seducer or member of the opposite sex hungry for affection.

The second point: Understand for yourself, and advise employees, that when the problem presents itself, it's necessary that one *do* something about it. Consider the situation carefully, seek the advice of a confidante if need be, and then take action. Do what Sally McAllister did when principal Lehman refused to take no for an answer: file charges.

Think through the possible personal and professional damage that may accrue from a more-than-casual friendship with a member of the opposite sex.

Report a sex crime — as Sharon King did not — to the police or school officials who will take action to make sure the aggressor does not victimize someone again.

Seek help. Seek advice. Be ready to maintain objectivity and rationality at a time when your emotions are racing to pull you in the direction of pointless paralysis.

Keep in mind and heed the words of Sharon King: "I've always said I was one woman who could never be raped . . ."

Chapter 6

"...She Wants Him So Badly..."

Mark Robards is in his late thirties. He serves as a field representative for his state's teacher association in the Southwest United States. He is active as a consultant to a state legislator and is often called on to testify before various state committees on education. Because these contacts often lead to a career in politics, Robards feels that his next professional step will be towards the position of a Congressional aide.

In terms of physical looks, Robards is more interesting than handsome. He dresses well. He is stylish and trim and his thinning hair is expensively cut. He has a quick wit, is well read, and is interested in a variety of subjects. He and his second wife have two children, twins, and he has two additional children from his first marriage. In his teaching days he was a high school social studies instructor.

The following is an interview — again, slightly fictionalized — with Robards concerning his affair with an eleventh-grade girl. The interview format, we felt, serves to provide the reader with authentic testimony from an educator who found himself in a situation like the one referred to in the rock song "Don't Stand So Close to Me" (see Chapter One). Rather than edit and summarize, we elected to present Robards' story direct from the transcript, only altering names and places.

Question: Tell us how the relationship began.

Robards: Sure. I had just come from teaching in an all-boys' school, and at a junior high school before that. I got this high school position in the middle of the year. It was located in Southern California, and it wasn't too long before we were in the middle of an early heat wave. The weather doesn't really have anything to do with what happened, but I always think of the hot spring weather when I think of Peggy. The heat set the tone, maybe, for some of the things that happened. I remember standing in my classroom door when I first got the job, right during the worst of the heat wave, and a beautiful young woman walked by wearing cut-off jeans and a bikini top. That was all. Talk about the ideal "California girl," she had long blonde hair and long sun-bronzed legs. It was that kind of school. Kids dressed like that, almost like in a stupid movie. I was *very* aware of the girls on campus. I wasn't blind. I was especially aware of them because I was rebounding from an ugly, ugly divorce.

Question: How old were you then?

Robards: I was in my late twenties. As I said, I was especially aware of the girls and they seemed to be aware of me. I remember one girl in class who stared at my crotch so directly that I moved from the front of the class and got behind my desk; her stare really unnerved me.

Of the girls that I first noticed, though, Peggy was not one. She was a teacher assistant — a service student — who helps teachers and gets class credit for it. I inherited her from the teacher I had replaced. She wasn't especially attractive in her face, but she had a fabulous figure. She certainly wasn't homely looking either, but she was not one of the classic "California girls" that seem to drive everyone, including me, especially including me, crazy. I guess I'd say she was very worldly, and during my free period when she was supposed to be helping me grade papers and whatnot, we talked a lot. She told me about her relationship with her boyfriend, and said they were very sexually active. I listened, and I tried to be sort of fatherly at first, but the more she talked the more I was interested in her and her body. I did not discourage this intimate conversation. In truth, I encouraged it because it was fun and sexy.

One day I noticed that Peggy was on the daily absence list, and was surprised when she showed up for her last class — mine. I asked her where she had been, and she didn't blush or beat around the bush. She had been at a nude beach with her boyfriend. That's when I became *very* interested in Peggy.

Spring break came and I had to visit my children. That's when the crazy thing of coincidence made me decide that sometimes fate is inevitable. It turned out that Peggy was spending spring vacation at her grandmother's — in the same town. She gave me the address, and as fast as I could arrange it I was there. I took my two kids with me, to give the visit some sort of respectability, I suppose, and we all spent the day going to the zoo and having a picnic. Strictly innocent. But that night it wasn't. Peggy came to my place and we got into some pretty heavy necking and petting, but no more than that.

Question: Did you think you were safe because it was another town? What went through your mind?

Robards: Thinking was never really a major part of the affair with Peggy. I was scared. I knew that it wasn't the sane thing to be doing. But when I wasn't scared I was horny. That I shouldn't be doing it registered all the time, but still I didn't have the feeling that I was doing anything wrong. I just didn't want to get caught. You know — don't *not* do it, just don't get caught.

After that fateful spring vacation I began to take her out at night. I kept telling myself this is crazy, this is nuts, but I couldn't help myself. Part of it was glands and hormones, pure and simple, but another part of it was connected to the stupid idea that I might someday die without seeing Peggy naked.

We often drove to a secluded park, just like high school kids, and we'd neck and steam up the windows. I'd pick her up after dark and a couple of blocks from her home. That went on for quite a while until I got up the nerve for the big move.

Near the end of the school year she broke up with her boyfriend and she came over to my home one afternoon after school and we made love. We got naked together, and part of me enjoyed it and another part of me loathed it because I was scared. That was the only time we made love while she was a student. But I knew she wanted the affair too. Like she told me she was on the birth control pill and that was her way, I figured, of telling me she was available — and willing.

But after the love-making I came to my senses, at least temporarily, and decided I had too much to lose. The affair was over now and that was that.

Question: It's interesting that you made the decision *after* the fact, isn't it?

Robards: Isn't it.

Question: How did Peggy react to your decision to end the affair?

Robards: I was surprised. She took it well. She took it in stride and that was that. I told her I didn't *want* to stop, that I enjoyed the afternoon with her very much, but I thought it would be better for the both of us if we didn't continue. She said okay. I guess she was ready to move on to something else whenever I was. She seemed to have a sense of satisfaction with whatever she was doing, as though whatever came next to her would be all right.

The next fall, her senior year, Peggy was a teacher assistant for me again. Nothing happened. Nothing. We were fine. I was in control, and I was also involved with a couple of teachers.

Peggy was worldly-wise. After she married, right after graduation, things didn't work for her and she divorced. After that we saw each other again, often. We became what could be termed intermittent lovers. She would come over and spend the night when she was between men and I was between women friends.

Question: There was never a concern during her senior year that Peggy might tell someone about your affair with her?

Robards: No. She was very sophisticated, let me tell you. I did wonder occasionally if she might maybe tell one of her friends, but if she did they were mature enough — or immature enough — to handle the news. I wasn't worried about her being indiscreet, which is maybe one of the great fallacies of having an affair. I figured she thought enough of me to avoid causing me embarrassment. That's probably whistling down a barrel, but in Peggy's case I was absolutely right.

Question: It seems impossible to think you weren't worried about being caught.

Robards: Nope. Never thought about it. Well, yes. Like I said earlier, I was scared, but I wasn't either. If anyone saw us in my car, I figured they'd think I was giving her a ride home. Maybe false courage, but I felt I was covered.

Question: Did no one of the staff observe the intimacy that was developing between you and the student and confront you with it? Wasn't it fairly obvious?

Robards: Never. I'm not sure that we were obvious. But that brings up a point about the school. You need to have a feeling for it to appreciate how I felt then, which was invincible. It was a very, very crazy place — it was very crazy and juicy. That's the right word: juicy. The principal was having an affair with the attendance clerk. Teachers were sleeping with students; teachers were sleeping with each other; teachers were even — get this — sleeping with the parents of some of the kids. I had affairs with four different women on the staff. It was incredible, now that I look back.

Question: What was the stance of the administration?

Robards: Prone, mostly. Are you kidding? That was one of the things that made me sour about administrators. I have since learned, of course, that there are good and bad administrators, but this principal was bad. The school was out of control. He was sleeping with the attendance clerk at the same time we were having chronic race riots. The whole district was a mess. At another school a teacher married a student in her senior year and nothing was done about it.

I got an excellent evaluation as a teacher and no administrator ever set foot in my class.

I probably could have — yeah, I probably *should* have been fired, but this was the kind of principal who'd stay away from evaluation in the classroom and then bitch to the guys at the Rotary Club about how he couldn't get rid of incompetent teachers.

Question: Might the principal have done anything to help you?

Robards: Certainly. I don't want to put the blame on him entirely and away from me, but I think he should have seen that I was fairly young, reasonably good-looking, and very single, and he should have advised me. He should have been very much aware of the atmosphere in the school, taken me aside, and given me some fatherly advice.

But the school lacked direction; there were no goals, no destination, no unification. That doesn't excuse what I did, but it gives you some perspective. There was nothing to lead me *away* from the attractiveness of Peggy, and everything was right to lead me *to* her. I know I was weak, even lecherous, but I was also without leadership or direction. A better administrator would not have let me slide into what I did.

Not that it ruined my life. As they say in soccer, no penalty, no foul. But I wish I hadn't done it. However, it made a kind of wierd sense at the time. The place was called the Country Club school and there was that feeling about it. The principal was a 'good old boy' and everyone's friend and the place was falling apart. My affair with Peggy was part of the whole picture.

I have since given some teachers the advice I wish I had been provided. I worked with a young guy who was a lot like me back then, and I pulled his coat and told him to be careful. A girl had complained to a counselor about his flirting, so I talked with him right away, told him to watch it, and reminded him that he was working with kids, after all, even if they did have adult bodies. I sure wish someone had given me that sermon when I needed it, though. I mean, Jesus, think of the image I had of the education profession then. I remember thinking what-the-hell, if I can get away with something this bizarre, what does that say about the leadership effectiveness of this whole damned shooting match?

Question: In your job as a teacher association field representative you now have to work with teachers and you defend them as an integral part of your job. Would you vigorously defend a teacher who was having an affair with a high school student?

Robards: Yes. I'd have to, at least to the extent to which his or her contract rights were concerned or involved. But not much after that. I would first advise the teacher to stop the thing immediately, to let it go. That's assuming no laws had been broken. I'd stick with the contract issues and then make sure the teacher quit.

Question: And if that didn't work?

Robards: I hate to say it, but I think the teacher should be canned if there is no resignation. *I* should have been canned. Teachers have a lot of power simply being an adult working with young people, and the power is especially strong if the teacher is charismatic. And good teachers are nothing if they are not experts at being charismatic. Teachers get a lot of power, and taking advantage of students sexually is an abuse of power when you finally get down to it.

These are kids we are dealing with, kids with adult feelings sometimes, and great bodies, but they are still kids. I had that brought home to me strongly when my oldest daughter entered puberty. It isn't fair for the teacher to seduce a seventeen-year-old because he or she didn't when seventeen and in high school. It's not right to try to make up for lost experiences when you're ten years older — that's taking advantage of the kids' lack of maturity.

I think I've become a good educator since the days of Peggy, and I'd say it's appropriate to nail people to the wall if they have more than a wild, one-time fling. I've had chances to have other student affairs since the business with Peggy, but I haven't. One has to draw the line somewhere, and I drew it back then when I decided that I couldn't keep up with her. I drew the damned line — partly out of fear, I admit — and I haven't crossed it since.

So, you have to get rid of teachers who take advantage of students in any way. You can't steer clear of controversies like my Country Club principal did, or it will sneak up and kick you in the ass. You're not avoiding it, only postponing it.

Question: In retrospect, do you think the affair had a negative effect on your teaching?

Robards: Not at all. Sorry. I was a good teacher and I stayed good. When Peggy was in class I didn't look her way. I didn't grade her papers one way or the other; neither harder or easier. I was very fair. She did her homework and I graded it the same as everyone else's. I had some kind of integrity when the bell rang to begin class. It was after the bell at the end of the day that I had trouble.

Question: What about her parents? You haven't mentioned them.

Robards: There's nothing to mention. I never saw them. She lived a pretty independent life, a life apart. I did meet them after she graduated from high school, when I was dating her as an adult.

Those kids at the Country Club lived a pretty strange style, like little adults with someone to pay the bills.

Question: Are you suggesting that Peggy seduced you?

Robards: I can't honestly say that, no. I'd be foolish to. I must have been giving out vibes that I was available, and she was a lot more worldly than I was, and it happened. She did some things in bed that I didn't even have the vocabulary, let alone the experience, to ask for.

The decision to get together had to be mutual, of course. But she set the atmosphere. I mean you finally make a pass at someone who is rubbing against you, not someone who is running away. And we were both rubbing against each other.

I mean she would touch me every once in a while, and she would — deliberately and seductively — show off her body when she was alone with me. Just by her posture and the way she took off her jacket or sweater was clearly sexual, clearly inviting. She could open a book in a way that would make a priest blush. I was weak enough or young enough or naive enough or horny enough to accept the implied invitation.

Question: Would you do it again?

Robards: No. I wouldn't. Admittedly, I'd like the experience of enjoying a body like Peggy's, but now it's fantasy, nothing more. A little fantasy now and then . . . what does it hurt? I've thought about doing it, but I've grown up. I've gotten over my youth, even though it took me more than thirty years to do it. I think that going to a junior high as my next assignment helped. I realized for sure that these were kids I was dealing with, and besides that, my own children were growing up. Soon my daughter began blossoming out, and I began to mature.

Question: What about love?

Robards: What about it? Love never entered the picture. I'm talking about sex, pure and simple. I've only been in love twice and I've married both women. But I've been in lust a lot. Love is a whole different thing. Sometimes I miss lust, but I've traded it for some other pleasures, and there is no comparison. The trade was well worth it.

Question: Are you saying you used the girl, then?

Robards: Sometimes I think so, but most of the time I think she used me. She was smart and sexual with a terrific body. I felt used by her. She knew what she was doing.

Question: What do you think you would have done if you had been caught?

Robards: That would have been difficult for me. I hope that I would have been honest and accepted the charges and the consequences without waffling. It would have been a terrific ordeal. My father was well-known in the area; he was a school board member in our home town, which wasn't too far away. Close enough that the newspaper served both communities. As I look back, I was worried that I could hurt some innocent people with the whole sordid thing. That was one of the things I worried about when I told her that we should call it quits.

But as far as getting caught, I didn't have a clue about what I'd do, I didn't have a plan. The only real thinking I did about it was to tell myself that it was crazy and I shouldn't be doing it.

Question: Any theories, other than what you've already said, about why you did what you did?

Robards: I don't know. I was alone. I was ready because I had just rebounded from a divorce. I seduced and I was seduced. But more than that, I was in a juicy, juicy school. The atmosphere was all part of it. I remember going to a graduation party that ended with a fight and required police attention. We were all drinking. Students, teachers, parents, relatives, little kids . . . and probably the dog and the cat. I ended up spending the night with some shirttail relative, a young woman (or an older girl, I don't know) whose name I can't recall. I dropped this little thing off at her parents' home the next morning and I never asked how old she was and she didn't take the time to tell me. It was that kind of atmosphere. The important thing to remember about this story is not that I took some young woman home for carnal and anonymous reasons, but that I went to a party as an equal, drinking, dancing and almost fighting with the best of them.

Like I said, the atmosphere was languid and sexual. The ambience was right. The kids were ahead of me and I was weak enough to lead and participate and follow and participate. I don't say that so as not to take blame, but I'm sure that was an important part of the problem, as was my own lack of will and responsibility. Part of me said that I was to die eventually and why shouldn't I have the rare pleasure of making love with such a sexual, lovely young woman? I can remember telling myself that I would be crazy to do it and crazier not to.

Question: If you had to give advice to someone in the first stages of the same kind of relationship, what would you say?

Robards: Don't do it. It's that simple. I know now that I was dealing with a child, even though she had an adult body. It's not in your own self-interest to get involved that way. People can understand that. That's easier to understand than ethics. It can create a lot of problems, so don't do it. I was lucky to get away with it.

Question: What if the person says "I'm in love"?

Robards: I'd tell him he's full of it. He's in lust.

Question: A woman?

Robards: The same, I think. Let me tell you this: a little later I had a student who was more attractive than Peggy, and she had the potential to be an exciting, interesting, responsive adult lover, just like Peggy. I could easily have fallen in love with her. I was teetering. She was gentle, quiet, smashingly beautiful, and obviously crazy about me. But I never did anything about it. It wouldn't have been right, let alone in my best interest.

Question: Has any guilt stayed with you?

Robards: Yes. I was hustled and seduced, but I was also a hustler and seducer. But that's not what the real issue is. I was supposed to be an adult. I could have hurt some fine people. My parents would have committed suicide. My mother still doesn't like the fact that my wives have been pregnant when I married them. No, I should have known better. But I sometimes wonder. If I was a stockbroker, a lawyer or a rock singer getting it on with a seventeen or eighteen-year-old girl that I met on a nude beach, I'd be a hero.

It wasn't really a violation of the girl, but it was a violation of

the trust that the parents give to the school.
I do feel guilty about that. I really do.

* * *

That concludes the interview with Mark Robards.
So why do educators fall in love — or lust — with students?
We will deal with that question in Chapter Ten. In the meantime,
Mark Robards' case serves to illustrate *how* it happens, and his
reflections after the fact speak for themselves.

Chapter 7

Teachers and Mature Students Revisited

Consider another slightly fictionalized case:

Rich Lawson is exceptional in the classroom. Last year he was chosen Teacher of the Year in your district and he was one of four state-wide finalists to be recommended to the State Superintendent of Instruction for State Teacher of the Year. One of the many reasons that he got that far was your sincere, warm, glowing and professional endorsement. Your superintendent is equally enthusiastic. Your terrific recommendation surprises no one. After all, you hired him from another district as soon as you were made a principal. You were both in the Peace Corps at the same time though you served in different countries.

Lawson is not especially handsome, but he *is* definitely charming and urbane. On the tennis court he looks better than he plays, but he plays well enough to beat you.

He gets a lot of respect in his class. He publishes poems now and then, most recently a love poem in a leading women's magazine. The school newspaper regularly mentions him in a friendly and respectful way as one of the most popular and effective teachers on the staff. Whenever you have follow-up evaluations with graduates and parents, they mention him as a model for a perfect teacher. They all say he is well-prepared, that he respects his students and that he has very high standards both for himself and for his students. A typical comment: "Mr. Lawson makes us want to do our best." Another: "I had a real advantage in college because of Mr. Lawson's class."

You have often said to fellow administrators that if all teachers were like Lawson, the school wouldn't need management.

But lately he has lost weight and has looked tired, and you have figured that he is having some trouble with his marriage of eleven years. You should know about it, but you don't socialize as much as you used to. *You* feel that *he* feels you've lost your

54

lust for life since you've become a principal.

You are genuinely surprised and dismayed when a parent calls to let you know that her husband saw Lawson and a student, Pamela Cortinelli, leaving a restaurant together. The restaurant was in a nearby, larger city. The husband also saw the couple kissing in Lawson's car in the parking lot.

You know that Pamela isn't even in Lawson's class because he's not teaching seniors this year. He wanted to teach remedial math courses where he felt he might have a more important educational impact. You tell the parent that there must be some mistake, but you will look into the matter and get back to her. You tell your secretary to have Lawson see you during his prep period.

You are anxious to talk with him because he is still almost a friend and you want him to know people are telling lies about him. You have a personal policy of discussing gossip and complaints with your teachers, but this is more than that. Your concern is more personal than professional. You again remind yourself that there is some mistake, but you have a sick feeling in your stomach when you ask yourself, "What will I do if it's true?"

Before Lawson's prep period, just by coincidence, you have a meeting scheduled with a mutual friend, the chairperson of another department. Your families used to get together often, so you ask in confidence how things are going for Lawson on the home front, adding, "He's been looking a little haggard lately."

The answer puts a nail in the coffin: "Didn't you know? He and Marcia split and she's living with another man. Rich has his own apartment now. She has the kids and he seems to to think that it's all for the best. So do I. I never did feel that their marriage was too hot, if you know what I mean. She used to begrudge the hell out of him for all the extra time he put into teaching. She wanted him to work with her in advertising, but he wanted to spend time in the classroom."

"Oh daaaaaaamn," you think as you wait for Lawson.

When you meet, he hammers in the rest of the nails and starts throwing dirt on the coffin.

"I know what you want to talk about. Pamela and me, right?"

Stunned, you nod in agreement and feel the weather change outside your window as he continues: "We're in love, deeply in love, and I don't know exactly what I'm going to do about it. We haven't slept together *yet*, and that's the truth, but I can't guarantee that for too much longer. We are definitely going to get married as soon as she graduates.

"I don't know what I can do to get this thing straightened out in my mind. It's the craziest and sanest thing I've ever been involved in. It's terrific. The same kind of excitement I felt when I went off to Africa in the Peace Corps."

You wince at that.

"I'm glad that you found out. I've got to get it off my chest. That's the only bad thing about it, the knowledge that I've had to keep it secret. Now I don't anymore. You know about it. That makes it perfect. I'm so relieved. You've got to help me work this out. You've got to be patient. God, I'm so glad that you understand."

Lawson's problem is the problem that we face here. What do you do in such a situation? What do you do when you feel that love is the factor and that the people involved are mature, possibly more mature than many other people you know who have forged lasting marraiges? Do you help?

Perhaps the most confusing set of circumstances for an administrator to face involves students and amorous teachers who have a sensible, understandable love, the kind that in any other situation leads to smiles from observers and long, shared lives for the participants.

This is a dreadful problem. It is fraught with danger. *Any* decision is bound to be bad. On the one hand, a capable administrator believes the old adage that a student is never touched in either love or anger, but, on the other hand, not even the most hardened manager can begrudge the cares of a couple who are magically and totally in love and on the way to marriage. Many of us just have to look a couple of generations and/or state lines away to see happy life-long relationships within our families with no different age spans than the Lawson-Cortinelli relationship under discussion here.

While it is difficult, if not impossible, to make a distinction between lust and love, let's face it, some times we have to do exactly that. We suggest that there are times when law and procedure might have to take a back seat to trust and the eternal cupid, but only a moment or two, mind, not for any longer. Give a few moments to sympathy and understanding when it comes to teachers involved with students in a genuine love affair. That is more than enough. You have the rest of your career to take care of. You have the rest of the school to worry about.

People do fall in love; responsible relationships develop and last. As we point out in Chapter 10, an administrator is hard-pressed to decide which is based on the lovestruck and which is based on the lust of an adult taking advantage of the gullibility and seducibility of a youngster, a youngster with little worldly experience.

We need to remind you here that the literary and the film stereotypes of the worldly, sexually confident teen-ager is a foolish one. It is created by wishful thinking from an immature 'adult' audience that is pandered to by greedy creators. And even if the sex-kitten dreams did exist with the force and passion that writers and filmmakers would have us believe, the public schools must still protect the young and must still keep the school free from sexual abuse. We are the good guys. Youngsters must be protected from preying or weak adults. We must all support that idea unhesitatingly.

This makes your decision a little easier. An administrator must always act on behalf of the total school. Guidelines have been offered to do just that. They are similar to the ones that have already been presented when it was suggested what steps to take initially when deciding how to act against a school employee who was clearly wrong.

The teacher's record, the student's age, the combined maturity, the presence of an adult advocate and the visibility of the situation are the major considerations here.

But, even though an administrator must weigh some crucial factors, it must be kept clearly in mind that the weighing in balance is only looking the other way for a moment. You are only considering a temporary truce. You are not considering whether or not to let the situation continue. That is not an option. You are only considering whether or not to give the two some brief thinking time before starting up the confrontation process.

As you decide this, the teacher's record must be considered. It is difficult to believe that a teacher who is into her third affair with a student — as was one woman we were told of — is ". . . really in love this time." She has a pattern that suggests someone somewhere along the line was remiss. A quick call to previous administrators about a teacher's past, discreetly checking with colleagues to see if there is any precedent for this kind of involvement, is a good idea. An administrator who is twice-burned is possibly once-compassionate and once-stupid. But more than that, a twice-burned administrator is certainly suspect in hindsight and in the glaring eye of the community and staff.

Consider an example:

Lew Whittier was a gifted art teacher in New England. His professional record was much like Rich Lawson's. Because of his work the high school was well regarded by East Coast art colleges. He sent much more than his share of students on to careers in painting and sculpture. Like Lawson, his students loved him. Nancy Morrow really loved him. Again, much like Pamela Cortinelli.

But there were some differences. There was no respect between the administration and the faculty, and Whittier had a 'health problem': Staggered by an ugly divorce — a Woody Allenesque escapade in which Whittier's wife left him for another woman — he was further knocked for a loop when his doctor told him that he was suffering from bone cancer. At least, that's what he told his few friends.

In his early forties, still healthy looking and handsome, still an avid jogger and skier, Whittier's teaching improved. He was cheerful and creative.

He jogged every morning around the school's track and soon Nancy Morrow was seen jogging with him. She was beautiful; she could pass for a thirty-year-old model anywhere even though she was just a junior. Her parents were alcoholic and pretty unstable. As one colleague put it, "In a way, she was a lot better off with Whittier than with them."

After his divorce, the regular habits of normal life were in disarray to say the least. He sometimes lived in his V.W. bus, sometimes on a friend's sailboat, sometimes in homes of friends when they were there or when they were on vacation. Only a few people knew of the chaos in his personal life because his school work was still exceptional. His principal, Edith Bluxome, who was near retirement and out of touch with the faculty, certainly knew nothing of his unusual life out of school. It was not really an important matter by itself.

No one was surprised by Whittier and Morrow's shared jogging because Whittier had an informally recognized reputation of 'being friendly' with attractive female students. But, the gym teacher who came upon them showering together in the coaches' shower room was a bit taken aback.

The gym teacher, you can bet, told his friends, but no one

told the principal.

Whittier had, though, told his principal about his bout with cancer. He also told her that he wanted to keep teaching as long as he could. Bluxome had tears in her eyes.

The lovers were caught in the shower again, and when one of the teachers told Whittier that he was going to talk to the principal with the story if something didn't change, Whittier said, "Hey, go ahead. I don't care. I love Nancy. She loves me. I've only got a year to go and I'm going to enjoy it. Besides, I bet you'd give a couple of years of your fat, stupid life if you could be doing what I'm doing."

The gym teacher didn't tell Bluxome, but a group of students did. They told her of rumors that Whittier and Morrow were not only jogging together, they were sleeping together in his bus and she was always hanging around his classroom. They didn't like it because teachers just shouldn't do that kind of thing, and, besides, it gave the school a bad reputation. Bluxome said she would do something about it.

She reluctantly called the art teacher in, and he quickly admitted it proudly, repeating in essence what he told the gym teacher, adding, "I'm not stopping, and I don't think we have much more to talk about. It's just between me and Nancy and that's that."

Bluxome did nothing. She explained that she was going to retire the year after the next and she was sure that Whittier's health would resolve the problem anyway. She couldn't bring herself to fight a dying man over murky issues about which she knew little. She knew, also, that Whittier was a formidable opponent and a histrionic faculty-meeting lawyer. She just didn't want the trouble.

Whittier continued dating Morrow through her senior year, though he didn't — as he had told friends he would — take her to the Senior Ball. His illness never took its toll. And the year after Nancy's graduation, he resigned to paint and sell real estate. Bluxome resigned the same year. Nancy Morrow lived with Whittier for two years until she left for art school in San Francisco. Rumors had it that he was back with his wife.

It is hard to say who suffered the most in this situation. An argument could probably be made that Whittier and Morrow probably look back on the whole incident with some pride and satisfaction. We think that the whole school was the victim.

Trust was destroyed between the staff and the administration. Though the affair was never brought to official view, it stewed under the surface. It was never brought to the faculty senate, the school board nor to any other faculty-administration group that functions in a school or a district. It never was brought out in the open; instead, it was discussed in bars and in commuter groups as just one more example of incompetent administration. The whole matter ran through the operations of the high school long after Bluxome's retirement. If she had looked at Whittier's record carefully, and if she had acted forcibly, she would have done her school a great service.

The age and the maturity of both people are paramount as one weighs options. But weighing options is only a prelude to how an administrator is going to squelch the affair in his or her school. Lawson showed admirable adult skills in his teaching, and — marital problems aside — in his personal life, at least as far as we know. As we find out more about Pamela Cortinelli, we see that she is an excellent student, one who is considered very mature by teachers and students. She is, though, very attractive and sensuous, the target of many male-faculty-room remarks. She was a class officer early in her high school career, but she quit to pursue local community-theater projects, and she was often mentioned as having great possibilities for a great career in entertainment.

If she were younger, or if she had a record of irresponsible provocative behavior, the administrator would have a clearer path, but she seems very mature for her age and she acts as an adult in most of her dealings with the staff. If you are an administrator, part of you may envy Lawson and his thrill of romantic, silly love. Given a girl-woman like Pamela, it is possible to believe him when he says he is crazy in love and he believes that he can form a solid marriage from all of this. And, besides, when you check her records, you find that she is eighteen and free to legally act on her own. She can write her own absence notes and you assume she can get married when and to whom she pleases.

But, still, you have to make the best decision for the entire school. Granted, Lawson and Cortinelli have a good chance to live happily ever after. Maybe. Maybe not. Whatever your appraisal of their chances, do not cooperate. Butt out. Do not offer any support. Hold back.

Say you decide that maturity and age are not a problem. If it were not for the problem of seeming to advocate sexual relations between students and teachers, you could let them go their own way. No way.

The advice and example of a man who married his student might be of value here.

Dennis Flaherty was a young, beginning teacher. Cheryl La Pointe was in one of his classes during his first year on the job. Only five years separated their ages. She was bright and energetic, much like Cortinelli and Morrow. Cheryl won the business department's award her senior year, her last in high school, Flaherty's first in teaching.

At the evening awards ceremony, Cheryl kissed him even though he wasn't the department chair who gave her the award.

The summer after graduation, because of Flaherty's recommendation, she got a job in a large accounting firm in which Flaherty was a part-time employee during tax-time. Much to his surprise, but probably not hers, they started dating. The high school faculty was young at the time — they'd dance together at the school dances occasionally and he took her to faculty parties, and within two years, they were married. Though they never dated while she was in school, and though they never had a serious relationship that went beyond the traditional one of student and teacher *during* school, they were soon romantically involved at a very close time to her high school years. When asked if he would have continued the relationship had it developed just a few months earlier, while school was in session, Flaherty now says, "Hell no. I'd be too frightened. They would have fired me on the spot. The school administration has to protect the students. I'd advise any administrator who finds a teacher/student relationship in his or her school to demand and put an immediate end to it."

Flaherty's marriage is now close to thirty years old, and it is still going strong. Cheryl moved up in the management ranks of a large bank and is now a vice-president in the Southeast. Flaherty is getting close to retirement; he is now working for his state's department of education coordinating state business curriculum matters.

Their story is one of success, yet the protagonist says he would recommend that the school move to squelch his relationship if it were to bloom on school time, even though he and his wife-to-be were mature and responsible.

* * *

An administrator must consider adult advocates in deciding between dramatically or subtly ending the relationship, the employment or the visibility. Does the student have the cooperation or the condemnation of the important adults in his or her life? If you feel that the couple is mature enough, you still have to check and see if there is any strong feeling in either direction by the parents. You must support the parents if they oppose the affair. You are not in the business of promoting marriages of any kind; you are in the business of educating and protecting children.

If a parent says their student is a child, you had better believe that student is a child. Never mind 'eighteen' and legal rights. Perhaps you might find a legal escape hatch. You could go against the parents' wishes if the student was over eighteen, or whatever the age of legal consent is in your state, but we strongly urge you not to do so, especially if you want to run a healthy, well-respected school. You are much better off taking the stand that you have to protect the whole student body and discourage the relationship.

We are reminded here of an administrator who was not enthusiastic about this book in its writing stage. He felt it would be inflammatory, that the public would misread it because, in his opinion, the problem was not too severe. When asked about some of the experiences he had gone through, though, he told of a young teacher who came to him and said that he was in love with a student and that he was going to start dating her. This administrator, who has a deserved reputation for being exceptionally supportive of teachers, said, ''You do and I'll have your ass fired.''

In several cases of the successful continuation of a student/teacher love relationship, the parents were supportive at best and resigned at worst. The parents concluded that the couple was bound to continue with or without their blessing. They chose to support or ignore the lovers rather than fight them, a much different situation than the one in which the adults are justifiably angry at the adult on your payroll who seduces youngsters.

You have to tell the cooperating adults that *you* cannot and will not cooperate, but you will not prosecute if the matter disappears from view.

Clearly, if the parents do not support the affair, it would be an unwise administrator who would put his or her interpretation of the problem ahead of the concerns of the parents of the student. When in doubt, side with adult advocates who wish to end the affair. When you believe the couple is mature enough to make it, and the adults are against it, side with the adults. When you are convinced that the lovers are right and that they have a great chance for success, still side with the opposing adults. If you have to make an error, make it on the side of caution, on the side of responsibility. Frankly, you have too much to lose and too little to gain by supporting the lovers in any case.

Love, of course, will find a way. It always has, but it won't find you a new job. Love might conquer all, but administrative leadership will not survive gossip and the community's lack of confidence where student/faculty personal relationships are tolerated.

We would much rather be considered harsh and reactionary by a teacher and his or her *paramour* than be considered unemployable by the school board. We all have enough trouble getting through the day without giving the community extra bricks to throw and topics to discuss in the supermarket parking lots.

As we mention in Chapter 10, it is important that *you* establish rules and guidelines. The only difference between how you handle a case based on love and one based on lust would be to give the lovers a chance to create a visible difference. If you can safely assure yourself that it is a love that will lead to marriage, or a modern version of it, then you can firmly tell the people that you will not work towards the dismissal of the teacher-half of the relationship, but you will be forced to do so, if the action continues to be or becomes visible.

You can then request the lovers to have an invisible profile, and to help them do that, you can help arrange a transfer to another school for one of the two.

Visibility and community knowledge are important factors here. These are pretty murky morals. We admit it, but we are simply saying that what *they* don't know won't hurt *you*.

Let us use a non-sexual example here:

Virginia Hewett took her assignment as a new principal of a large suburban high school. During her first week she toured the campus, and in the custodian's office and work room she found a printed sign that said, "Obviously you want someone down the hall. You've mistaken me for someone who gives a shit." She laughed at the sign, and then she asked the custodian to take it down. He said that it had been up for two years. "What's the matter? Don't you like my sign? The teachers love it."

Hewett answered, "To tell the truth, I think it's pretty funny. I just laughed, didn't I? But funny doesn't have anything to do with it. It is not appropriate. How can we ask students to be respectful of adults who are offended by their vulgarity if we don't censor ourselves? It is wrong for us to display that kind of language in front of teen-agers."

"That's hypocritical bullshit!" he said.

"Not at all. Leaving it up would be hypocritical bullshit. I'm not above using profanity, as you shall see, but there is a time and place for it, and I don't expect adults to swear in front of students and that's that."

Hewett's point is well taken in this context. We cannot in any way visibly condone a sexual — or, if you prefer, a 'romantic' — relationship between students and teachers. It is too confusing to the students, teachers, community and parents. Not only would doing so tell the students that we would let the teachers take advantage of them, we are telling the staff and the parents that we will allow students to take advantage of employees.

Do *something*! Even if it is wrong. Neither you nor your school can afford to let a situation that involves the loaded area of sex impinge on the school day. You have enough trouble with budgets, buses and basketball. A teacher dating a student, no matter how idealistic or platonic the involvement, is purely and simply not acceptable. We don't care if you have an adolescent Mother Theresa taking tea with a pedagogical Jimmy Carter *sans* lust in his heart. The community feelings, the clear and consistent taboos, the inherent need for sexual protection of the young, all make it absolutely essential that you give no implicit or explicit sanctioning to any sexual or *quasi*-sexual or potentially sexual contacts in your school. You need to keep the school free of this kind of gossip, to keep the school running efficiently, to keep your own career on the track and, also, most important, to protect students and teachers.

You need, though, to have some kind of Solomon-like ability to sense the depth and maturity of the people involved, so you can give them at least one shot of advice. You need to know somehow that the relationship will in fact end happily. This is no easy task. Who among us can make this kind of conjecture about the *regular* marriages that we face on normal days? How could you ever figure out what happened to your close friends, let alone two people with whom you have not shared deep friendship and long nights, one of whom is still legally — and if not physically, probably mentally — a child?

* * *

In summary, one final word about looking the other way: Don't! Imagine a situation in which you decide to ignore a liaison between a teacher, one, say, like Rich Lawson with whom we opened this chapter. You begin to notice another teacher — one of those marginal ones who is not bad enough to fire, but who is not good enough to teach *your* children — is getting a bit cozy with a cheerleader and you begin to pick up some gossip. When you confront him, he will probably say, ''You didn't stop Lawson, did you? Everyone knows you don't care about the kids. Why pick on me?''

It won't be too long until the superintendent talks to you about your evaluation schedule.

You must examine the teacher and the teacher's professional record and past record of relationships with students. You must examine the student's motives and maturity. You must talk with both parties and the parents and you must abide by the parents' wishes, except if they wish to encourage the couple. Take no part of that deal. You have to — above all — decide what is best for the school in the long run, not what is best for the student and the teacher who are in love. Their love is their problem, not yours. Considering all things, you are a school administrator, not a marriage counselor or a marriage broker.

Chapter 8

Rape Prevention

In the early fall of 1983 two girls left the campus of Hinkley High School in Aurora, Colorado, to have lunch at a nearby fast-food restaurant. There they met two young men driving a car with Nebraska license plates.

The girls struck up a conversation; the boys said the car was for sale and asked if the girls would like to test drive it. They decided they would.

They finished lunch and hopped in the car. With one of the girls driving, the boys directed them to a deserted horse corral in a desolate farm area east of the city. There, both boys took turns raping one of the girls and preventing the other from escaping. They then drove off, leaving the victims at the scene.

The girls made their way back to school on foot, reported what had happened, and received immediate attention and assistance from the nurse, counselor and principal. The incident was never reported in the media, and the police never found the young men or the car with Nebraska plates. The parents of the girls expressed deep appreciation for the manner in which the school personnel helped their daughters, and it was never suggested that the school was in any way at fault. The girls, all agreed, had simply behaved foolishly — had erred tragically.

Why relate the unpleasant tale if it was not school-related? For two reasons: first, to point out that rape may be a problem in your local school, if not sooner, probably later; second, to illustrate that even when school officials can't prevent the crime of rape, they *can* and *should* have a program to provide instant support and sensitive assistance to victims. Such was the case for the two girls from Aurora, and the prompt, professional help from the school staff was invaluable to them and their families.

Further, it needs to be emphasized that *where* the crime occurs is irrelevant; the victims — male or female — need a support system in the public schools. The crime could have occurred just as easily on the school campus as in the country-side. That it did not was simply a quirk of fate.

Before proceeding, let's agree that rape is a crime of violence rather than a crime of sex, and let's agree that the primary focus of any discussion about rape is on men attacking women. However, keep in mind that rapes of men by women also happen, albeit less frequently, according to the experts.

(Surprising? Perhaps, but Dr. William H. Masters of the Masters and Johnson Institution, and Dr. Philip M. Sarrel, associate professor at Yale University School of Medicine, agree that men and boys are sexually assaulted by women more than is thought possible, and since men are just as loath to admit being raped as are women, the extent of the crime may never be known with any accuracy. Masters and Sarrel identify four categories of rape by females: 1) forced assault (rape); 2) the seduction of a boy by a female babysitter, housekeeper, or tutor — recall Angela White and Tom, presented in Chapter Two; 3) incest; 4) aggressive sexual approach to an adult male by a dominant woman who intimidates or terrifies the victim.)

Rape is a crime of violence, and it needs to be understood that it is even more heinous when the crime is committed at school. As has been made abundantly clear throughout this narrative, we believe school should — *must* — be a safe place for youth, a sanctuary from the violence of the real world. In truth, however, it is not.

Consider: In California alone, in 1981, there were 668 violent sex offenses committed in the schools, according to figures published by the state's Department of Education. In the same year, 598 violent assaults were directed against certificated school personnel in Los Angeles.

Just one rape, especially one in a school, is one too many. Violence against any staff member or student needs to be avoided. School is not a place for mindless terror; teachers and students deserve to be protected. Unfortunately, that protection all too often does not exist for school people. They are victimized by the same twisted forces that attack in our neighborhoods, streets, alleys, bars, family gatherings, shopping centers and parking lots.

A complex problem that goes from incest to date-rape to gang attacks, rape is the forcing of unwanted sex on another person. It is usually violent, and it leaves both physical and psychological scars in its wake. It is anathema to education. The rape of a teacher has an especially emotional impact on a school. And, contrary to popular opinion, you can do a good deal to prevent rape on school campuses and you can do much to alleviate the problems related to rape if and when it does happen.

At the risk of belaboring the point, it needs to be emphasized that rape is a shattering, degrading experience that will, if not dealt with maturely and compassionately, have a deep and serious impact on the victim's life. A teacher, we suggest, is even more vulnerable than other members of society. A teacher is to be respected, to have safe status in our society. Though we know that is not always the case, we believe in particular that the women who teach should be protected from the cruel forces of physical violence. That is not to say we recommend knights in armor be assigned to roam the halls to protect the maidens within the castle, but it is to say that we do respect teachers in the abstract, and we do as a legacy of our childhood give a special place in our spiritual hierarchy to the women who educate us. It's the same *more* or cultural expectation that causes men to fight to protect their mother's name. It's doubtful that any of us pictures the teacher in the movie "Looking for Mr. Goodbar" when we reminisce about our favorite elementary teachers.

Raped teachers report a disabling experience which is further complicated by their concern about how their students may view what happened. A raped teacher has to face her class again, which may be teeming with insensitive youngsters. The insinuations or cruel observations will not all come from the students, of course. For example, the character in Sonia Wolfe's novel about the rape of a teacher, *What They Did to Miss Lilly*, is asked in the faculty lounge why she was dumb enough to let a thing like that happen to her. Rape victims are all too often made to feel they are to blame, as if it is their fault they were victims, as if they did something that caused it. Again, recall the comments made by Sharon King in Chapter Five, the teacher who was raped by a fellow teacher and couldn't tell her husband or the authorities for much the same reasons: "I've always said I was one woman who could never be raped . . ." But she was, and it was years before she could talk about it.

In terms of our schools, it seems clear that a crime of the magnitude of rape should be given as much serious attention as a fire. All schools have systematic fire drills, but how many are ever really evacuated because of flames? Schools have exercises for earthquakes, tornadoes, and floods. Likewise, schools should have workable plans for preventing the occurrence of violence in general and rape in particular.

Schools are a microcosm of society. As Mary Conroy suggests in an inservice videotape on rape prevention, prepared by the San Diego County Schools in California, in this day and age we all need to be a little paranoid. Our schools are not safe; even the best, with campus monitors and burglar alarms and district security offices, are not one hundred percent trouble-free.

As an example, consider Linda McGinnis, an attractive elementary teacher who elected to work late in her classroom one afternoon. The building was empty except for a secretary in the main office who could be contacted by intercom. Linda, in truth, was alone in her part of the building some distance from the office. When trouble arrived, Linda had to activate the intercom switch to call for help — it was a switch she was unable to reach.

A man, unfamiliar to Linda, entered her unlocked room and said he was a parent of one of her students. She accepted the statement (it may be argued that most teachers are an unsuspicious lot) and began chatting with him. Without thinking, she turned her back to him to get some papers from the desk and he grabbed her from behind, forced her to lie face down, then told her he had a gun and he wanted her money.

"Take it," she said immediately. "My purse is in the closet on the top shelf."

When the man made no move to get it, she knew she was in for serious trouble. The struggle was violent, but the man raped her and escaped. No one heard her cries, and of course the intercom switch was in the off position.

Linda McGinnis' ordeal might well have been prevented if school officials had established a few simple rules.

It *is* possible to lock the barn door before the horses are stolen. It is only necessary to think about some preventive steps and then be firm and realistic enough to consider that violent crimes and sexual assaults *can* happen in our schools and it's possible to be prepared. It *is* possible to plan intelligently in order to thwart thugs and rapists, and it's just as possible to provide support that will lessen the trauma of being attacked if and when rape does happen.

Here are some simple guidelines:

1. Become aware of dangerous situations, potential trouble spots in the building and around it;

2. Alter those dangerous spots to eliminate the potential for trouble;

3. Provide inservice for staff and students about what to do, how to protect themselves when it's possible and appropriate;

4. Develop a plan to provide victims with considerate, compassionate support

The following information and examples will help illustrate how one can implement the above guidelines.

1. Be Aware of Dangerous Situations.

Two men, Rory Elder and Glen Scrimager, who work for the California State Department of Education on a special project that focuses on crime in the schools, state that they can determine immediately the anti-crime status and attitude of any campus the minute they arrive. They know it is high if they are met and confronted by adults who ask them their business in a friendly but firm manner, or at least ask politely if the strangers need help or directions.

Conversely, Elder and Scrimager can tell just as certainly that a schools' discipline and security are weak if they are not challenged when a staff member spots them on the grounds for the first time. Being challenged, they agree, is a sign that the people in that school care about one another.

Simple, yes, and if your school (and district) does not have signs on all school doors directing visitors to check in at the office and state the nature of their business, and a staff of teachers and custodians alerted about how to confront strangers, then by all means implement such a system directly. Not only will this procedure help screen out folks who should not be there, it will help prevent not only rape but kidnapping as well — and the incidence of divorced parents coming to school and kidnapping their children is also on the increase.

A school that is responsibly but not fanatically on the alert, that inservices the entire staff to care about all the people associated with the school, is one that will have few problems. The most sanguine administrator knows that the additional effort pays dividends. Being alert and being determined pays off. Are teachers instructed to turn the intercom button on when they work alone in their rooms after the day has ended? Are people advised to travel in pairs to cars or bus stops when the sun goes down early in the winter? Do teachers feel the need to follow a strange group of boys to an isolated lavatory or do they ignore them and head for the coffee room? They are educators, yes, and not policemen, true, but the vibrations of their trained antennae are invaluable in helping break up a possible drug deal and/or avoid a mugging or rape. It is reasonable and necessary, really, to have the entire school staff as alert to trouble at school as they are alert about locking their cars and dwellings by habit.

Dangerous situations exist in every school. There are portable classrooms located out of sight in remote corners of the campus; there are teachers who like to stay late and work alone; there are students who linger after school every day; there are parents who threaten violence; there are graduates who keep returning for no apparent reason (except perhaps the favorite female teacher they come to visit is especially attractive); there is an ex-boyfriend who didn't like taking 'no' for an answer. School people should not panic about these situations, but they ought to know how to recognize them and be ready to get involved and learn how to get out of them or get them resolved for the safety and welfare of all concerned.

School administrators need to encourage staff to invest several pounds in prevention in order to get back tons and tons of cures.

Administrators need to ask staff to bring dangerous or unsafe situations to their attention so solutions can be found. Principals need to set a tone that allows staff to bring such matters to them. It's helpful to ask the police to assist in inventorying a building for potential problem areas, just as is done with the fire department when inspecting for potential fire hazards. A free and safe environment requires constant vigilance.

2. Correct the Danger Spots and Problem Areas.

Once a problem area has been identified — a dark hallway, a poorly lighted parking area — do something about it.

It cannot be emphasized too much that once a problem has

been brought to the attention of the officials responsible, it can't be ignored. A somewhat different example may bring that point home to administrators who tend toward apathy when action is required. A teacher aide in a Midwestern school complained that she got severe headaches, a sore throat, and a mild skin rash every time she used the spirit duplicator to run off tests and worksheets for teachers. She asked for gloves and better ventilation in the work room. Nothing happened. A short time later she filed a Workmens' Compensation claim, contending that the ditto machine work was damaging her health. She had a physician's opinion to back her.

As the arbitrator of the claim pointed out, the principal had been made aware of the problem and ignored it. The investigation that followed her Workmens' Comp claim verified that ventilation was inadequate and there were no gloves available. The district settled with the teacher aide for ten thousand dollars and felt thankful to get off that cheaply.

Once the problem has been identified, it's imperative that something be done to at least *try* to correct it.

If a female secretary is required to work late and alone, it's only prudent to make certain someone is there to meet her and walk her to her car.

If Linda McGinnis had been required to lock her door when working alone and had let no one in without calling the office first and/or leaving the intercom on, she likely would never have been raped.

If a hallway is identified as too dark to be safely travelled at night, get it lighted or mandate that an alternative route be used.

Finally, work routinely with situations that can be easily and readily influenced, and that's most often the staff and their attitude of awareness and caringness for one another and the children. Administrators can create a climate of caring whether the building is in the ghetto or plush suburbia.

3. Provide Inservice for Staff and Students About What to Do.

The potential for serious crime varies, and therefore the extent to which school administrators plan preventive inservice — and the topics of the inservice — will vary.

A few years back the principal of a large, urban high school in Arizona was confronted with a deadly serious problem with teen gangs. The boys' gang went by the name of the S.M.F. which, the principal stated, stood for "Savage Mother Fuckers." Their girl friends established a support gang and called themselves the R.W.B. — "Rowdy Wild Bitches." That year the S.M.F. and R.W.B. gangs terrorized the school: there were assaults, fights, vandalism to cars and the school building, even an aborted attempt to burn it down.

In that school, while it may be considered controversial, an inservice program to teach the staff rape prevention, including tactics for fighting back, was perfectly in order. Some might argue that encouraging physical retaliation is tatamount to escalating violence. The administrator and his or her staff must decide, but it can be argued that doing nothing adds up to acquiescing because of fear. If victims — or would-be victims — choose to be passive, that's their option. We argue only that the inservice should be offered; then let the staff make the decision.

Self-defense and rape prevention workshops are recommended for school staffs. Mary Conroy, mentioned earlier, offers workshops in self-defense where participants learn how to kick kneecaps, pull testicles, and gouge eyes. Brutal? Yes. Chilling? Again, yes. Scary tactics not for the squeamish, but certainly self-defense methods that give the potential victim a fighting chance to control and perhaps succeed in the battle with an attacker. Victims may choose to submit rather than fight, to give in to rape on the assumption that the assault is preferable to being maimed, crippled or killed in the effort to resist. In any event, they have been provided with alternatives, and the decision is theirs.

The San Diego County Schools' program for self-defense and rape prevention is excellent and is available for schools that wish to adopt it.

Rape prevention programs are also recommended for students, and at the elementary and junior high (or middle) school levels it is also recommended that school officials develop and implement a "How to Deal With the Bad Stranger" program.

An excellent 'bad stranger' program model is available from the Davenport (Iowa) Community School District. It was jointly developed by school officials and the Davenport Police Department.

4. Develop Plans to Support Victims.

Should all well-intentioned plans for prevention fail, schools should have a program available to assist the victims of rape.

First, the plan must be underpinned by the understanding that the blame for rape must never be placed on the victim.

"What were you doing in the car with those men in the first place?" would no doubt be the reaction of many who read about the two girls from Hinkley High School mentioned at the beginning of the chapter. To ask the question is to place the blame for the rape on the victims, and that is not right.

"What do you expect, the way *she* dresses?" is a remark that unfairly blames the victim, implying she invited someone to violate her sexually. Untrue and unfair.

The plan to assist victims requires a team of staff members who understand the need to be sympathetic to the victim's physical needs and psychological needs as well.

It is recommended that schools identify two or three staff members to serve as the support team, and then have them work with the local rape crisis or rape intervention team to develop a plan and program.

Chapter 9

Sexual Harrassment

The headline in the October 23, 1982 issue of the *Des Moines Register* was a charitable understatement: "Ex-Superintendent Admits Unprofessional Conduct."

The school superintendent, a married man in his mid-forties, had attempted to kiss and fondle seven female teachers over a two-year period, had asked them for dates, had made sexually suggestive remarks, and on one occasion exposed himself.

Few would argue that the superintendent's actions constituted sexual harrassment, and even he admitted the improprieties when the local teacher association blew the whistle. His actions, according to a psychiatrist, were motivated by severe stress and a not-so-latent desire to destroy himself. In terms of his career, he succeeded. As a result of his harrassment activities, he resigned his position and the Iowa Department of Public Instruction accepted the 'voluntary surrender' of his professional certificate.

The Iowa superintendent's case is reasonably open and shut in terms of harrassment. However, it is not always as clear-cut. Consider the following example:

Jeanne Gregory, secretary to the superintendent of a large, urban school district, had been asked to bring some budget information into a cabinet meeting of four male administrators. The issue at hand was the serious business of budget reductions, but the men were joking with one another and Jeanne. As the superintendent put it, "Sometimes we joke and get a little crude in our remarks when things are tense. It's a form of venting the tension, I guess."

No real argument with his explanation, but the 'venting' may have resulted in sexual harrassment of an employee. How?

As the meeting progressed, it became evident that some of

75

the data Jeanne Gregory had prepared was incorrect, incomplete.

"Looks like you screwed up," one of the administrators said, laughing. "Jeanne, you've been had."

"Yeah," she said, a little embarrassed. "Sorry about that, but some days I can be had for a quarter."

The administrator took a twenty-five cent piece from his pocket and flipped it over to her. "Your place or mine?" he asked.

It was a seemingly harmless incident, but was it also sexual harrassment? If so, who was harrassing whom?

Jeanne Gregory was asked that question. "No," she said. "We were just joking. I consider that sort of thing — light humor with maybe a little sexual innuendo — to be a fun part of this job. I meant nothing, and neither did he. The thing with the quarter brought a lot of laughs and diverted attention from the fact that I had not done the job correctly. In fact," Jeanne concluded, "I could tolerate a lot more of that kind of harrassment, if that's what some call it, because it helps lighten the sometimes dull work."

Sexual harrassment, which some would argue had happened to Jeanne, is truly in the eye of the beholder.

For example, according to an Associated Press article by Kay Bartlett, published in 1983, the Working Women's Institute, based in New York, defines sexual harrassment as "any unwanted attention of a sexual nature from someone from the workplace that creates discomfort and/or interferes with the job."

For Jeanne, the incident with the quarter and the "your place or mine" remark created no discomfort. For another secretary, it might have been very distressing and upsetting.

Sexual harrassment, then, which may range from an unwanted remark to the violence of rape described earlier in Chapter Five, is as real and prevalent in the schools as it is anywhere else. It touches teachers and administrators, male and female alike, just as frequently as it does students and parents, and dealing with sexual harrassment can be both difficult and emotionally draining.

If you are inclined to dismiss casual remarks such as the one made to Jeanne Gregory as nit-picking, or to conclude that any female who is offended merely lacks a sense of humor, don't.

There is ample evidence that sexual harrassment is a part of the fabric of society and it thrives in education. Can any school employee argue that none of these activities exist within his or her particular school system: 1) generalized sexist remarks (*a la* Archie Bunker); 2) inappropriate and offensive but essentially sanction-free sexual advances (such as placing one's hand on another's lower back or other 'unsafe' touching area); 3) solicitation of sexual activity or other sex-linked behavior by promise of rewards (such as a perfect test for sex favors described in Chapter Two); 4) coercion of sexual activity by threat of punishment; and 5) sexual assaults.

The National Advisory Council of Women's Educational Programs estimates that ten to twenty percent of female students have at some time encountered sexual harrassment.

Admittedly, the statistic is an estimate. Research undertaken for this book does not help verify it, but certainly many examples of the five 'harrassment categories' were readily available and some definitive guidelines emerged.

Consider, for instance, the fairly open-and-shut case of Meggie Glass, a freshman at a university in Michigan. Meggie entered an elevator in the education building along with several other students and a custodian. At the third floor, everyone exited except Meggie and the custodian, John Gage.

The door closed and Gage turned to Meggie. "I like your sweater," he said, reaching over and placing his hand on her breast. "You're good-looking, sweetheart. Mother Nature was good to you."

Meggie pushed him away, but was too terrified to speak. The elevator stopped and she rushed out. John Gage followed, saying, "What's the matter, don't you like dirty old men?"

Distraught and frightened, Meggie darted into a graduate assistant's office, burst into tears, and related what had just happened. The graduate assistant reported the incident, and Meggie subsequently filed a complaint against Gage.

Two weeks later, following an investigation by university and union officials — marked by Gage's denials and conflicting explanations for what happened — the university fired the harrassing custodian.

Gage grieved his dismissal, but he didn't win. A simple guideline for handling incidents of sexual harrassment was evident in the opinion handed down by the arbitrator who heard the case: "I am persuaded to the facts as testified to by Meggie

Glass. It is simply not credible that she would manufacture such a tale out of whole cloth. . . . Significantly, she was so distraught as to break into tears while reciting the facts . . . such emotional outburst also lends credibility to her version of the facts.''

The guideline that emerges from the arbitrator's judgment is clear: report an incident to someone in authority, and tell it like it is.

So how do you go about making certain that incidents of sexual harrassment get reported? Define it in your teacher handbook for each building and ask principals to discuss it in faculty meetings. Acquaint them with the five 'activity categories' presented earlier in this chapter. Have them advise teachers to be alert to the problems and ready to report an incident when they encounter one.

Then be ready to take action. Have a plan, even if you later have to modify it.

Is this guideline so obvious that it doesn't merit emphasis? Some might think so, but there is plenty of evidence that victims of sex in the schools all too often do not report or complain.

Why on earth don't they, one wonders. Fear? Perhaps. Confusion? Shame? Maybe excitement. One can only speculate.

Parents, teachers, students, administrators — all need to understand and emphasize the seemingly obvious: victims of sex offenders *should* report incidents of harrassment immediately.

It is a simple guideline, but as is usually the case with simplistic rules, there are related problems. Things are never that simple after all.

Therefore, parents, teachers, students and administrators need to know that there are four *caveats* in regard to the guideline:

First, some victims will never report an incident of harrassment (and you're stuck with the rumors);

Second, when an incident is reported, authorities do not always act on the complaint;

Third, some 'victims' use the reporting of an alleged incident as a not-so-subtle reverse form of sexual harrassment;

Fourth, failure to act on a complaint can land the person who received it on the sorry end of a court judgment and fine if something isn't done about it.

The examples that follow illustrate these guidelines.

1. Some Victims Never Report Their Problem

Sharon King, the elementary teacher whose case was cited in Chapter Five, was raped by another teacher. She never reported the crime, and one has to admit that her reason for not doing so was fairly credible. Sharon represents the victim who will never report an incident of sex harrassment, even a crime as violent and humiliating as rape.

2. Some Authorities Won't Act on Complaints

The second example — where an allegation is reported but nothing is done about it — comes from New Jersey.

Mrs. Gail Lowenkopf was convinced that the vice-principal of the school her twelve-year-old daughter Becky attended was sexually molesting the girl.

"Becky spent more time in his office than in class," Mrs. Lowenkopf stated. "She always had two or three dollars in her purse when she came home every day. Where did she get it? I hadn't given it to her."

Becky, according to her mother, was both a liar and a manipulator, and she liked sex. " 'I'm not going to make love to you,' I heard her tell a teacher in that school," Mrs. Lowenkopf said. "The implication I got was that she would make love to someone, then, and she admitted to me that she let the vice-principal touch her. But she wouldn't admit to anything else."

Mrs. Lowenkopf thought she had enough information to file a complaint; she was deeply concerned and went to the principal of the school. "He told me it was nonsense, that Becky was simply an office assistant and that's all there was to that. He refused to listen. So I went to the superintendent. Nothing. I even went to the police. Everyone said I had no evidence, and Becky refused to say a word. But I know that man did bad things with my daughter, and maybe two other girls."

When no one would investigate the situation for her, and when her daughter came home one day and told her she had spoon-fed her lunch to the vice-principal 'because he's so good to me,' Mrs. Lowenkopf removed her daughter from the school and enrolled her in another.

3. Allegations That Are Sexual Harrassment in Reverse

The third example — where the victim files a complaint that can't be verified and it results in damaging another's reputation — comes from the Rocky Mountain West.

Jerry Lehman, the young, single high school principal mentioned in Chapter Five, romanced Sally McAllister, a guidance counselor on his staff. The relationship faltered and subsequently Sally filed harrassment charges and destruction of property charges against Lehman, and the local newspapers had a field day with the story.

Lehman, who may or may not have been guilty of harrassment, was now himself being harrassed.

4. The Consequences of Not Acting on a Complaint

An example of the fourth guideline — what may happen if a complaint is filed and the person in authority decides *not* to act on it — occurred in 1982.

Two parents came to the office of elementary principal Bill Gardiner and told him that his third-grade teacher, David Kent, was molesting girls in the classroom. They alleged Kent had touched the vaginal areas and chests of eleven different girls in the class.

"Frankly," Gardiner stated, "I didn't believe it. I considered the parents to be exaggerating tales their daughters had told them. They were very emotional, almost hysterical. David Kent is a good man, a close friend, and I couldn't believe it."

Gardiner did nothing. He stuck by his convictions, but it was an error he wishes now he hadn't made.

The parents went to the police and filed charges of child abuse against the teacher, and the police in turn filed charges against Gardiner for failure to report the alleged child abuse.

"If I had believed that Kent was sexually molesting girls," Gardiner told the judge at his trial, "he wouldn't be in the classroom. He'd be in the morgue."

A firm and noble statement, without a doubt. However, the court ruled that while Gardiner may have owed some loyalty to his teacher, he owed a higher duty to the children. He could not be judge and jury in these matters. Gardiner was found guilty and given the maximum fine. Kent, who pleaded innocent, was scheduled for trial. He was tried nearly six months after his principal was found guilty and fined, and interestingly enough, Kent was found innocent on all counts.

Gardiner was right, then, but so was the judge who admonished him to follow the law and not take it upon himself to be the judge and jury.

The potential for allegations of sexual harrassment is immense. The cases presented here substantiate that people in the schools are not immune from becoming victims.

As reporter Ann Bartlett pointed out in her syndicated article for the Associated Press, an invitation to dinner can become an invitation to a lawsuit if the relationship sours, as it did in Jerry Lehman's situation.

Following the guidelines presented in this chapter will afford most adults in authority some protection, however.

Furthermore, the Mrs. Lowenkopfs in our midst may profit from the lesson of the Gardiner-Kent incident. If the parents cannot obtain satisfaction from the school authorities, the avenue of filing a suspected child abuse complaint is guaranteed to produce an investigation. *That's the law*.

The issue of sexual harrassment is growing. It may be as difficult to avoid becoming a victim as it is to avoid a flu epidemic. It may be inevitable. The best preventive, then, is awareness.

One needs to understand how widespread is the problem, and to be on the lookout for dangerous situations, and to be prepared to act prudently. Educators need to be alert to the necessity of keeping the sex-neutral relationship of teacher/student and counselor/client undistorted. An unwelcome, non-reciprocal emphasis on the sexuality or sexual identity of the student by the educator constitutes sex harrassment; it is a distortion of the neutral relationship demanded.

Students need to be informed about their rights and the channels for lodging complaints. Teachers — all educators on the staff, really — need to be sensitized to the parameters of sexual harrassment. All education institutions need to develop formal grievance procedures, if none exist, to protect students from retaliation, and to assure that appropriate sanctions are taken with the offenders.

For parents, teachers, and school administrators, the choices can and will be difficult, unpleasant, even painful. But the choices must be made with careful thought, with measured courage, and with the advocacy of the child foremost in mind.

Chapter 10

Why Teachers Get Involved

That teachers become attracted to students is not surprising. Neither does it stretch our understanding of human nature when adults entangle themselves with members of the opposite sex and it's clear they should not. On the other hand, we are taken aback when teachers — anyone in education — commit deliberate, observable, irresponsible actions because of that attraction.

Just as we can understand some larcenous joking among secretaries as they handle the gate receipts from a huge crowd at a high school football game, we are begrudgingly tolerant of the lounge chatter about the sexual attributes of a school's girl-women. Most male administrators have either participated in or observed ribald conversations about the sexual allure of some particular female student. No doubt the administrators are happy that parents aren't privy to these exchanges, but nonetheless the conversations are seldom discouraged. Sexist? Probably. So be it. Men talk about women.

Women, it is noted, seldom engage in the same kind of open speculation, for whatever reasons.

Lounge chatter about sexy students may not be professional, but it is understandable. The attractiveness of young women is obvious, and our culture reveres female beauty and youth. We are confronted constantly with beautiful females who possess fine physical attributes and are of indeterminate age. Television, from commercials to football games and their cheerleaders, would be barren without them. Their presence is just as prevalent in America's schools.

Those who enter our schools frequently remark about it. One visiting poet, for example, offered the following: "I can understand being attracted to students. The girls are amazingly beautiful. Even the eighth-graders. They flirt with me and I sort of flirt with them, but I know enough, like most people . . . if it goes

83

beyond flirting it will be harmful.''

The poet's comment sums up the most common attitude about the proper distance that needs to be maintained between adults and students. Yet, very obviously, some adults go beyond flirting. They cross over the line and break the taboo, both men and women.

Why?

Why do some people act, while others are content to dream and fantasize about what might be but must never be?

One reason, clearly, is that our society confronts us constantly with the temptation. Sex and youth sell. Attractive young men and women of poise, beauty and vitality reflect the what-ought-to-be. We diet, we take drugs, we jog, we invest fortunes in creams, cosmetics and clothing to be eternally young and handsome. We are compelled to do so because our people are as dedicated to staying young and virile as Hitler was to his blond, blue-eyed Arian Master Race.

We think of sex and youth a very great deal of our time because we are continually bombarded with the glories of sex and youth in our daily lives — the magazines we read, the newspapers, advertisements, television, movies, novels, music. It is, very simply, a stable part of the American Dream. Right or wrong.

By contrast, consider an anecdote related by a friend who recently visited the country of Turkey in search of antiques for his business. One of the Turkish shopkeepers, he said, remarked that a serious problem for him was the German, English and American women who came into his shop in abbreviated clothing. Every once in a while one of the workers would emit a low groan and go after a particularly scantily attired female tourist. The other men in the shop would have to scramble to keep him in control. In our mind's eye we can understand why a man or woman, unaccustomed to seeing so much exposed flesh, might take a risk for such a lovely prize. People who dress provocatively do indeed provoke. For some reason, we don't care to acknowledge that honestly in America.

We seem reluctant to understand that a male teacher finally may be as overwhelmed with lust for a teen-age school girl braless in a tight blouse as was the shop clerk in Turkey.

That point acknowledged, we still are left with the fact that the majority of the adults in education manage to teach without developing a compulsive attraction for the students in their care.

Again, why? It is not within the scope of this book to provide a definitive answer to the question, but neither is it a question we choose to ignore. Psychiatrists and other professionals in the field of mental health can undoubtedly probe the issue and provide better answers, but in an effort to help school administrators and parents deal with problems they encounter, we offer some food for thought.

We will sidestep the incidents where it appears that sexual harrassment or assault results from mental abberation. The superintendent in Iowa referred to in Chapter Nine, for example, who was motivated, according to one psychiatrist, to commit inappropriate acts because of stress and a desire for self-destruction. His case is similar to that of a junior high principal in the Midwest who pinched female teachers and felt their breasts because, in his attorney's words, he was under severe mental stress. We don't pretend to be able to analyze these convolutions of mind and character — pleas of temporary insanity, if you will — with any degree of success.

However, with the reader's indulgence, we present a "Why Theory" comprised of three elements or dimensions: Venial, Lustful, and Romantic.

Let's begin with the Venial Motivation, the easiest to recognize. Recall your religious education or your vocabulary assignments: a venial sin is one that is pardonable. If one commits a venial offense, one gets in *some* trouble, but it can be forgiven if one plays his cards right.

The largest number of sexual harrassment complaints fall into this category, and they are easily nipped in the bud. Like a timid base runner, most teachers can be brought back into line with a good eye — knowing the pitcher (in this case the principal) is watching them — and a respectable reminder now and then.

Often teachers (usually male teachers, please note) will let slip casual and very off-color comments to students who wear revealing clothing, or who are sexually precocious. These teachers may say something inappropriate to an entire class, something smutty, something in the vein of locker room humor. We're not talking about teachers who use profanity in front of students; that's another matter. We're focusing on the teacher who makes reference to sex, uses double *entendres*, and tells occasional blue stories. This person is not to be confused with the teacher who uses a literary work that contains sexual scenes or references. Unless the teacher has a consistent habit of introducing literature featuring explicit sexual material, he or she is not included in this discussion.

We are talking about the leering educator still behaving too much like an adolescent. The reason for his or her venial behavior is fairly clear: the titillation is an end in itself, and talking sex is safer than doing it. The behind-the-barn tickly danger of being a bit of a rake is its own reward.

These adults get a childish kick out of an off-color joke or flirtatious remark. It brings them satisfaction. To discourage the Venial Sinner, an administrator need only point out to the offender that while the joke or remark is relatively harmless, nonetheless it is completely inappropriate and it must stop. The matter is closed. Once the offending teacher knows that the comments have been noticed and labeled offensive, the teacher more often than not will cease and desist.

Sometimes venial comments and cute flirting remarks filter up to an authority in the school because they are not so cute and are not considered harmless. When this happens, the principal has to determine if the comments and parries represent probes in disguise, efforts by one party to explore the possibility for positive and intimate responses. The remarks, in other words, represent a form of emotional radar. Will a student react in a way that could open the door to a more intimate comment or action? Again, the sensitive administrator must assess the track record of the teacher, the nature of the comments, and the degree of offense taken by the person or persons registering the complaint.

Emotional radar operators are prone to engage in flirting that can lead to trouble. There are handsome, attractive teachers of both sexes who can and do use their good looks and charm with ease — in faculty meetings, at cocktail parties, and, unfortunately, at school. When they do, the result is usually a student with a crush on a teacher. While most educators discourage or ignore infatuated students, some choose to encourage. They need the admiration, attention and esteem; it reinforces their egos and builds self-concept. The danger seems to escape them, but it is there. In most cases everyone weathers the platonic student-in-love-with-a-teacher storm. However, the administrator and parent must monitor and be alert and be prepared to issue firm reminders about a teacher's responsibility as an adult. It is not an easy task, nor is it often a comfortable job.

Two case histories — one about a verbal Venial Sinner and

another about one whose manner of dress set off emotional radar beams — and a description of how they were handled will serve to specify the degree of confrontation required to alter the behavior of those who would flaunt their sexuality in front of students.

The first example involves Hal Wilson, a California high school photography teacher who possessed classic good looks and an equally classic flair for the double *entendre* and flirting remark. "Let's go into the dark room and see if anything develops" was one of his favorite remarks reserved for the more attractive girls in his class. "I've got twelve inches, but I don't use it as a rule," was another.

The females in Wilson's photo course weren't exactly complaining, in the opinion of a counselor, but they did let the counselor know that he made frequent sexual innuendoes to them. The counselor, a good friend of Wilson's, tried to be helpful: "Better cool the remarks with the girls, Hal. They may start complaining to someone who has more clout than I do. It's no big deal right now, but they could make it one."

Wilson, already bitter about being transferred to the school against his wishes, did not take the advice kindly. "What big deal?" he retorted. "My remarks are no worse than how they talk to each other. Except they talk dirtier. Hell, what they see on TV and in the movies is a lot more vulgar than anything I've ever said. These girls are on the make, and sometimes I wish I could get in on the action. And besides, half the time *I'm* offended by what *they* say."

The counselor shrugged it off. The warning had been delivered. Parenthetically, though, it's worth noting that the counselor would have been well-advised to alert the administrator, because in very short order the principal, Jeff Jackson, paid a visit. "I've gotten a parent complaint about Hal Wilson," Jackson said. "You heard anything? This father says Wilson is making suggestive remarks to his daughter and he's ready to punch him out if it happens again. He also said the girls talked to *you* about the problem and you did nothing, you're protecting Wilson. What's going on?"

Belatedly, the counselor confirmed the girls' accusations, apologized, and principal Jackson proceeded to process the complaint. A check with Hal Wilson's former principal revealed that there had been no similar complaints about Wilson in the past. Jackson concluded that his photography teacher was guilty of making cheap remarks for their thrill value . . . an offense in the Venial Sin category.

The confrontation between principal Jackson and Hal Wilson was swift and to the point. Wilson attempted to defend his remarks as he had with the counselor, but Jackson made certain his teacher got the message: the remarks to the girls had been made, they were inappropriate regardless of any reason, they were not to be made again. "It doesn't matter what the students say or how foul-mouthed you perceive them to be," said Jackson. "Your job is to correct them if it's needed, not join them. What *you* say to students is my business and yours, and we're the professional staff. Make certain the sexual innuendoes stop."

They stopped.

The second example deals with one Mrs. Marcia Leonard, a new addition to the guidance and counseling staff of a junior high in the northwest section of the country. Marcia, too, was beautiful and youthful; one of the tenets of her philosophy included the decision not to wear a bra.

Larry Cornelison, assistant principal of the junior high, was made aware of the situation — which may not be a direct Venial Sin problem, but certainly borders close enough — by one of the secretaries. "Mr. Cornelison," the woman said, "I don't think I should pull any punches. Ms. Leonard is doing a pretty good job, but I have to tell you that I hear the boys talking about her not wearing a bra. It may be none of my business, but I don't like hearing the youngsters joking about it. She *does* have an ample . . . ah, well, the boys say if it's a cold day or the air conditioning is on, one of *them* could poke your eye out."

Cornelison had to suppress a smile, and assured the secretary that he'd take care of it. In truth, Cornelison said he didn't have a clue as to what he should do.

He assessed the situation in his mind. The decision to wear or not to wear supporting undergarments was the lady's, he reasoned. Calling 'official' attention to her bralessness might create more of a problem and cause Women's Liberationists to descend upon him. Was Ms. Leonard coming to work *sans* brassier to excite young men, to lure them or seduce them? No. Marcia Leonard, he knew, lived with a handsome local attorney and the chances of her seeking the sexual attention of twelve and fifteen-year-old boys were nil. Besides, Cornelison was aware of the

Shields vs. Household Finance decision, and he knew that the courts had ruled that one's personal life outside the office has no real bearing on one's performance on the job.

Was she dressing provocatively to gain attention? Was it a symbolic or crucial statement she felt she needed to make regarding the role of women in education? Was it, perhaps, just more comfortable to not wear a bra?

Cornelison didn't know, nor did he know just how he should go about bringing up the subject.

As Cornelison thought about how to confront his counselor, he stated, he also worried about possible repercussions. He had vivid memories of the public scalding another principal, now retired, had received at the hands of the local press when he insisted that one of his teachers could not wear mini-skirts in his school. Cornelison didn't want to be tarred with *that* brush.

However, he couldn't practice avoidance. He could hope Ms. Leonard would just magically appear at work properly attired, but that was too much the head-in-sand approach. He was prodded into action when he discovered graffiti and a crude cartoon drawing of Ms. Leonard, the anatomy of her chest explicitly rendered, in the boys' restroom.

He called her to his office for a conference, and tried to summon forth everything he'd learned in psychology courses about reaction-formation, defense mechanisms, and the subliminal gymnastics the human mind performs when one wants to do something but is afraid to follow through. Why worry? said a voice in his head; the way she plumps out a blouse is pleasing to behold. Forget *that*, said another voice. She has to be told that her appearance is distracting and hurting her effectiveness.

He decided to direct the conversation toward solving a problem, and to avoid saying anything that might be taken as an inappropriate accusation. "This is going to embarrass me as much as you," Cornelison said to open the conference, "but I think you need to know how some of the students — the boys, especially — perceive you. They joke that you don't wear a bra, and . . ."

Marcia Leonard's arms folded protectively across her breasts, startling Cornelison. He glanced out the window and continued.

". . . and the boys say things. And I hear about it, and it may be uncomfortable, but I think we shouldn't ignore it. You should know. The boys tell jokes and make crude humor. That concerns me, as it probably does you, too.''

Cornelison had played his hand correctly, and with sincerity, and it got results. Marcia Leonard was responsive. ''You know,'' she replied, ''my boyfriend and I talked about it this morning. He said it was no one's business, but I *haven't* felt good about it. I appreciate what you're telling me.''

''Well, I have to confirm your thoughts,'' Cornelison said. ''In education, we have to realize that we're hired to help youngsters, not add to their problems. You need to counsel, and you need to decide whether or not the sexual tension you create is making it difficult to do your job.''

Cornelison was relieved when Marcia Leonard thanked him and said she would think over his advice. He was more relieved when she reported to work the next day wearing a bra under her sweater. His conference about venial transgression had been successful.

The step over the line from a venial sin to an act of lust is a short one. It is not possible, unfortunately, to recognize any one pattern of actions that will identify the adult bent on seduction. The emotional radar beams given off by those whose intentions are labeled wrong or evil by society don't look any different from those of the person who intends no harm.

The *why* is difficult. Why are there adults who use their status as educators to make sexual treaties?

It appears the forces that create sexual deviancy are as mysterious as they are compelling. However, in pursuing our ''Why Theory,'' we'll attempt to examine the elements and dimensions of the Lustful Adult.

What could have motivated Stephen Adams, a fifth-grade teacher in Colorado who was honored by a local service club as ''Outstanding Young Educator'' in 1976, and recognized by the local newspaper as ''Public Servant of the Year'' in 1972, to seduce three of the boys in his class between the years of 1978 and 1982? Adams, an eighteen-year veteran teacher, was judged to be an outstanding educator by administrators and parents alike.

''He was like a father to my boy,'' said the mother of one of Adams' victims during the trial, ''and that's why he should go to jail, to show my son that you can't do something wrong without being punished.''

The mother of another boy Adams had assaulted was equally

devastated. Her son told her he had been sexually molested by Adams ten times over a period of four years, beginning in 1978. The boy ended up in a mental health center with severe identity and personality problems.

Tragic, yes. However, as the judge in Adams' case stated when he meted out a three-year prison term: ". . . Tragedy is tossed to the wind when teachers, who have such a very special place in a community, admit to harming a child. Word of such harm ripples through a community, and when this type of conduct is involved, the rippling is like a wave. Repeated conduct over a span of several years . . . make that rippling deafening in its intensity."

The outstanding teacher and community leader, Stephen Adams, went to prison. Why? Why did he sexually assault the boys?

Perhaps his brother saw a reason. Stephen, he said, was extremely religious, lived with and cared for their mother, and was probably a virgin who would never marry. Those add up to fairly substantial elements descriptive of a lonely person in need of affection and sexual gratification, who finally succumbed to the many pressures best described by psychiatrists.

The desperate loneliness of Stephen Adams very nearly generates a degree of sympathy for the sex-offender, but the feelings of pity are diminished significantly, if not totally, as one surveys the damage he inflicted on three innocent youngsters.

Allen Green, on the other hand, represents a lustful teacher apparently motivated by ugly, evil forces that stir not pity, but absolute contempt, and almost defy explanation.

Green was a business education teacher in a U.S. Territorial School in the Pacific. Unlike Stephen Adams, Green was considered a mediocre teacher. His evaluations were lukewarm, but he was not judged to be poor enough to warrant dismissal. It was not his competence that was at issue when news began to filter in to his administrators about his extracurricular activities. Shortly after Green's wife left for an extended vacation on the U.S. Mainland, rumors began to crop up about wild parties at Green's home involving G.I.'s and students.

After a boy came home very intoxicated, and his father went to the school to seek help in finding out where he'd been to get himself in such a condition, Green's principal began investigating rumors that led to the discovery that Allen Green was not only organizing parties featuring marijuana and alcohol, he was accommodating sex parties as well. For a price, it was alleged, Green was arranging to provide the soldiers with sex, and the prostitutes were high school girls. The principal was able to prove to his own satisfaction that Green was pimping; he confronted the teacher and fired him. His contract was revoked and he was flown back to the United States on the next plane. All of the facts surrounding Green's case have never been revealed. The administration's effort to keep the lid on the scandal was successful, but enough is known to conclude that Allen Green was sick. His mind was twisted and he had no concept of morality as it is normally understood in education. Regardless, he lost only his job, and was never prosecuted or referred for psychiatric evaluation.

Again, we consider the question: Why? Why would any person who chose the teaching profession end up pandering sex to make money? Why would that person host alcohol and drug parties for minors, students from the work place? When a person abuses the institution that exists to educate and protect rather than victimize, we not only ask why, but we become outraged as did the mothers of the boys who were violated by Stephen Adams.

One finally comes to the conclusion that it may not be possible to determine why there are Fagins in the world; only that it is clear they are there.

Because the line separating the venial sin from the dimension of lust is narrow and easily crossed, those who lead schools must be alert and purposeful. Rumors must be diligently tracked and resolved; truth must be found; it may never be presumed that an allegation of lust is too preposterous to merit concern. It may never be possible to really understand why the *id* becomes more powerful than the superego and the crime is committed. It *is* possible, though, to understand that it happens. Believe it and be ready to investigate the charge.

Examining the third dimension of the Why Theory, which deals with those whose relationships blossom within the Love or Romantic dimension, is taking a look at what has confounded even the poets, let alone scholars and newspaper columnists who dispense advice to the world.

How does one explain love that develops between a teacher and a student?

How does one explain love, period?

"True love," that physical attraction leavened with mental compatibility and characterized by commitment and responsibility, is far more mysterious and inexplicable than is sexual lust. Packaging the ingredients of love in a myriad of settings and arrangements has been the bread and butter of playwrights, artists, and novelists for centuries. The standard give-and-take of courtship and dating among young adults who assess and bargain their desires and dreams for the future is magical, frightening, dull, exciting, and about as easy to explain as it is to nail smoke to the workbench. Love stinks, according to one song writer. Love is beautiful the second time around, says another. Love is blue . . . Love makes the world go 'round . . . Love is . . . .

You supply the ending.

At its simplest level, love is highly complex. It is at one moment exactly like sexual lust, and the next moment it is very sweet and entirely different. Lust ends in climax; love continues through morning sickness, debts, success, failure. It endures.

To the point at issue, love develops between teachers and students. The love in question rises above — transcends, if you will — the dimensions of venial sin and lust. It works. It clicks. The couple live a happy life in spite of the fact that their love began and was nurtured under the disapproving, reproachful eye of society.

Why is that and how does it happen and what advice needs to be considered by those who must handle the situation?

Think over the cases presented in earlier chapters, and then add to them the interesting perspective of John Collins, a high school English teacher who posed this thought: *why not?*

John Collins stated for the record that he fell in love with a girl in one of his English literature courses, Anna Clements, in the late Sixties. "I was married then and I still am," said Collins, "to the same woman. I don't think our marriage is much stronger today than it was then, and that was pretty rocky. But we tolerate, we exist. Perhaps that had a great deal to do with my love for Anna Clements. I spent a lot of time thinking and brooding about my unhappiness, and how wonderful it would be to have a wife like Anna. But she was one of my students."

Collins loved Anna from a distance. "I never dated her, never kissed her, never said a word to her about my feelings, but we both knew," he said. "Now, almost twenty years later, we run into each other frequently and the electricity is still there. She's in the school business too, at the central office in another district, and every time we're together her eyes say 'why not' to me, and I'm sure mine read the same. She is in her mid-thirties, I'm forty-five; she still attracts me, even more because her marriage failed and she's raising her son alone.

"Why not? Why didn't I? I still love Anna, and the way she hugs me when we see each other tells me it's mutual. But I was afraid to do anything about it then, and I guess today I've concluded it's too damned late. It would probably hurt her."

John Collins' declaration supports the contention that genuine love carries with it the desire to act decently and to be protective. He found himself charmed and in love with a girl who was, at the time, eight years his junior, and he was not willing to risk his career, her career, his marriage, her future . . . but their desire to be together, he contends, is still strong.

Albeit the John Collins' of the world may be in short supply, his interview and candid opinions lead one to speculate: how many men and women in education fall in love with students but keep that love in the closet and go about life as though it didn't exist? Again, why?

The 'why not,' or 'why didn't I' attitude of Collins is worth sharing, because it illustrates the fact that there are people in education who have held their emotions in check, but — to resort to a somewhat trite expression — it's very likely they are bombs waiting to explode, accidents waiting for a place to happen. The frustration of Collins is of nearly twenty years' duration. It's very likely, even highly probable, that the bitterness will not remain under the surface forever, particularly for those whose marriages are unhappy. It appears to the authors that Collins is a fine example of someone about to erupt into what has been popularly labeled a 'mid-life crisis.'

How many others share his status? How many more times must he encounter Anna before he decides to step back and take a stab at rewriting history, at reordering his life? Will it be with Anna, or will it be with one of the young girls now enrolled in his English classes?

John Collins was very open, very willing to talk about the love he concealed but never gave up. That's worth remembering, for the administrator: a confidential conversation with a staff member may be very revealing, and may be just what the administrator needs to assess the potential for problems and consider what counsel and advice might be preventive. When a principal suspects that love is possible between a teacher and a student, it's time to exercise personal judgment. Talk to the teacher. If it appears appropriate, offer advice and spell out options in a non-threatening posture. Those who are genuinely in love will likely listen.

However, to return to our opening statement: it is part of human nature that persons will entangle themselves with members of the opposite sex when it's clear they should not. Therefore, be ready to accept the reality of your advice going unheeded.

If the action or entanglement is in the Why Category of the venial sin, you act firmly. If lust motivates an act of sexual assault, you again act firmly in behalf of the victim with the knowledge that the results will be tragic and scarring for one or both parties, and you'll be stepping carefully with the law and the courts at your elbow. Finally, if genuine love is the reason why a teacher becomes involved with a student, you confront, you advise, and you monitor. The relationship may end happily, as attested to in the cases presented in Chapter Three. And, of course, it may not. But concerning yourself with the why of the situation will help you decide which way to act.

Why do teachers fall in love with students?

You decide. Your guess is as good as ours, and now you know that understanding why — if you can determine the why — will help you steer your course of action for what you will do about the teacher in love with a student.

Chapter 11

Epilogue: Being Prepared

It's clear by now that the problem of sex in the schools, as well as approaching those who would choose to taste of the forbidden apple, is a many-splendored thing. Exactly how school authorities decide to deal with a given situation involving sex in the schools is in itself very situational, as has been amply demonstrated in the ten preceding chapters.

When the problem is a teacher and a minor student, the steps to be taken are reasonably clear as set forth in Chapter Two: consider the age of the child; determine if there was an eyewitness; is there a confession; look for physical evidence that logically leads to the person responsible; hope for the involvement of an adult advocate for the child, usually the parent; then act. Keep in mind the concept set forth in several earlier chapters: when in doubt, it's smart to file charges of suspected child abuse and let the police and social services agencies enter the investigation.

Remember that the use of a polygraph test, if legal in your state, can be very helpful and effective in determining guilt or innocence.

It's important to keep uppermost in your mind that schools must be safe places for children, and that children have the expectation that adults — especially teachers — will protect them. It is equally important to know that in spite of this, and despite tough laws on the books against sexual relations with children, there is an epidemic of sexual abuse of children in this country, in the words of Dr. A. Nicholas Groth of the Connecticut Correctional Institution.

We'd like to underscore too the fact that most pedophiles — those who seek out children for sexual purposes — are men, but there is increasing evidence that many are women; furthermore, rape is generally a crime against women by male attackers but females also rape men and boys.

If that isn't contradictory and muddlesome enough, add in the point that pedophiles often convince themselves that they are doing the child a favor, that they are providing love and affection the child needs by using them for sex. Convoluted logic indeed, when it's evident that society takes a very different view, that their actions represent taking advantage of the child's feeling of being unwanted or unloved or vulnerable and confused.

Finally, keep in mind that when a solid case has been established against an educator who victimized a child, it's inadvisable to make the charge against the teacher "immorality." Stick to the specifics, which will usually add up to a violation of a law, board policy or school rule. The concept of "morality" tends to change with the times.

When the problem is a staff member and an older student (sixteen years and up) the guidelines change a little, primarily because the student may be a very willing love partner and not at all inclined to see himself or herself as a victim. Still, the administrator must act, as discussed earlier. It's helpful to understand one additional guideline not mentioned earlier: an administrator may pursue a dismissal case and be successful — even if the employee is judged innocent in court — if the administrator can show that the staff member is no longer effective in his or her job because of the charges. In short, it is possible to argue that publicity, electronic media coverage, and/or the hue and cry of the community is so loud that the employee is rendered ineffective.

Two cases, one mentioned in the Introduction and David Kent's situation in Chapter Nine, represent how it can happen, even though they were not cases of teachers in love with older students. The music teacher mentioned in the Introduction chose to resign, and Kent — in the midst of a great deal of sensational publicity — was non-renewed because he was not on tenure and therefore could be terminated without cause. The point here is that if they had not been removed as they were, good cases could have been made to the effect that their ability to resume their work and be successful had been destroyed.

When the student has attained the legal age of consent, things get very difficult. In addition to advice previously offered, we have only one additional suggestion to contribute, and it comes from an unusual proposal made at the University of California at

Berkeley in 1983. The faculty there proposed that any 'romantic or socio-sexual relationship' between professors and students be outlawed. Noting that there were several dozen student-teacher sex relationships annually on campus, a committee chaired by history professor Richard Abrams called for the sex ban and asked that the faculty behave as professionals. Ignoring the old adage that 'You can't legislate morality,' the school's Academic Senate passed the resolution by a vote of 20-14.

It may eventually become necessary to make similar campus rules if what Harry Zehner said is true: "From a purely logistical viewpoint, student-professor romances are inevitable." Zehner is a college professor who fell in love with one of his students, eventually married her, and wrote about it in *Cosmopolitan* magazine ("Love and Lust on Faculty Row," April 1982), from which the above quote was taken.

When the romance is between staff members, heed the advice presented in Chapter Five: step in and act quickly, transfer one of the parties if it's possible; provide some plain talk to the entire staff about the community's and district's views about faculty romances; and file charges if it's appropriate.

Bear in mind, though, that filing charges, or even having absolute knowledge that the party or parties were guilty of a sex taboo, doesn't necessarily mean they'll get the ax. Can a teacher be fired for having sexual intercourse with another man's wife (she was also a teacher) in the back seat of a car (particularly when the woman's husband is hiding in the trunk of the car)? Yes, one would certainly think so. No, said the Iowa Supreme Court *(Erb v. Iowa State Board of Education, 1974).* The court ruled the incident was unlikely to have an adverse effect on the erring teacher's effectiveness, since the sex tryst happened away from school and at night and was an activity of his private life; he was reinstated.

No matter how steamy, outrageous, or bizarre the matter of 'immoral behavior' may appear to you, if it is confined to an educator's private life, then the legal concept of *nexus* must be satisfied. It must be proven in a court of law that there is a connection between the conduct or behavior of the teacher or administrator and his or her fitness to teach or administer.

As readers well know, when an issue ends up in a court of law, the answer all too often ends up being both Yes *and* No, depending.

There are no guarantees.

When the problem is sexual harrassment, we have nothing further to add beyond the guidelines and policies recommended in Chapter Nine.

In conclusion, please understand that *why* professional educators break the taboo is impossible to pin down. Might it be linked to a 'mid-life crisis'? A divorce? Stress? True love? The teacher's traumatic childhood? Just plain lust?

You decide. Better yet, invite a psychologist or psychiatrist to kick around the question with you for an hour or so and it will probably still come out the same: your guess is as good as anyone's; you decide.

What we'd like you to remember is that it *does* happen, and you need to do something about it. Hopefully, this text has provided some insights and guidelines that will help you when a problem with the forbidden apple for the teacher pops up in your school or district.

ORDERING INFORMATION

If you are using a borrowed copy of *The Forbidden Apple* and would like to order a copy of your own, please send $13.95 to:

ETC Publications
P.O. Box ETC
Palm Springs, CA 92263-1608

There are no shipping charges on prepaid orders. California residents, please add 6% sales tax (84¢).